Also My Journey

Also My Journey

A Personal Story of Alzheimer's

Marguerite Henry Atkins

UMW 88

MOREHOUSE-BARLOW

WILTON

DEDICATED
TO

My beloved husband, Dick (Richard F. Atkins),
who taught me much of laughter and love, and
of the gentle grace of living, and dying, with God.

"That I May Trust" on page 83 was first published in *The Living Church* (Milwaukee, Wisconsin) January 25, 1981. Later, it was given a musical setting by Thomas Matthews and published as "Open Mine Eyes" by the H. T. FitzSimons Co. (Chicago, Illinois) in 1981.

Morehouse Barlow Co., Inc.
78 Danbury Road
Wilton, Connecticut 06897

ISBN 0-8192-1362-4 (cloth)
ISBN 0-8192-1385-3 (paper)

Library of Congress Catalog Card Number 84-62378

First Printing October 1985

Printed in the United States of America

Foreword

"Also My Journey" is a moving account of a man's medically incurable disease and of how his wife coped, by the grace of God, for almost fifteen long years with an agonizing situation. But it is more than this: it is the story of a couple who loved each other very much, and loved God even more.

In my work in the healing ministry, I meet hundreds of people each year, and cannot possibly remember all of them. I met Dick only once and very briefly at the healing mission Marguerite describes, but I never forgot him.

Even at that time he was in the clutches of Alzheimer's disease, but this was not yet evident to the casual observer. As we shook hands after the service that night, I saw only a gentle man with a zest for life—a man in whose face shone the love of God.

Marguerite tells their story honestly and eloquently. Indeed it was her journey as well as Dick's, and perhaps even more so, for much of the time he was, mercifully, unaware of what was happening to him.

Much of the time Marguerite was under my spiritual direction, and as one crisis after another asserted itself with Dick, I watched her meet each one with courage and gallantry. She was not particularly strong physically, and I pled with her again and again to conserve her own strength; to take less frequently that long, tiring drive to see Dick. But she persisted. She was a marvelous wife to Dick, who was ill for more years than they had enjoyed a normal marriage. She left no stone unturned to assure him the very best care he could receive, both medically and spiritually.

I do not for one second believe that the dreadful disease from which Dick suffered, was the *primary* will of God. However, although His primary will was circumvented, the offering to God of Dick's illness and her own anguish, was honored by Him and used for His glory.

I share Marguerite's conviction that God used her husband and his life to serve as an inspiration to others, manifesting until the end, and despite his physical and mental deterioration, the love of God. Dick's spirit, which never ailed and was always whole, touched many lives, especially the patients and hospital personnel. All felt their lives enriched by their contact with him.

Marguerite's courage; her love of God and for Dick, were likewise an inspiration to all who knew her and were aware of what she was enduring. She assuredly had my admiration from the beginning to the end of Dick's ordeal which was also hers. The way she handled their situation should be of great help to anyone—man or woman—who finds himself or herself with a spouse suffering from Alzheimer's or any other long-drawn-out, so-called "medically incurable" degenerative disease.

For those who are healed by God, we offer praise and thanksgiving. For those like Dick, whose illness God used so beautifully, we also praise and bless His Holy Name.

The Rev. Emily Gardiner Neal, Deacon

A Personal Note

from the Episcopal Bishop of Southwest Florida

For the space of ten years I served as rector of St. Luke's Church in Fort Myers, Florida where Richard and Marguerite Atkins were active communicants. Following Richard's declining health and ultimate hospitalization, I was made Bishop of Southwest Florida and therefore did not have the opportunity to see him in the Arcadia Hospital as often as I otherwise would have done. I attest to his patience, his faith and his acceptance of his suffering in heroic fashion. His death, after those many years, was to me the ultimate healing.

Marguerite Atkins has distinguished herself in terms of her spiritual insights and literary skills. Whether in poetry or in a book or in simply a meditation, she reveals an intimacy of relationship with God which is most rare and appealing. I commend this writing to everyone in the sure knowledge that each person who reads it will find immense personal edification, especially in the author's authenticity, that most rigorous kind of honesty involved in this presentation.

I pray that this book may be widely distributed and joyfully received by those who would find new meaning in the pathway that leads to God.

February 12, 1985
†The Rt. Rev. E. Paul Haynes

Contents

Prologue

Beauty Is the Hem of God's Own Garment

"Beauty is the hem of God's own garment"
Look quietly and intently for a while;
Fragile things that are so very delicate
Are often those most favored by our smile.

Lovely things in any form or color
Delight us as we go upon our way;
So it is that we're most apt to worship,
It's easy then to turn to Him and pray.

But, storms are beautiful the same as flowers,
The stones that cut our feet, He made them, too:
Waters rough are part of His own beauty,
And woodlands dark are worth our struggling through.

Beauty *is* the hem of God's own garment,
Let us touch it, let us hold it as we go;
The moonlight only comes to us in darkness—
But darkness is not dark with Him, you know.

One

The Deepest Bond

A Thing of Beauty

"A thing of beauty is a joy forever,"
A talented one once said—
But "beauty's in the eye of the one who beholds"
Is one other thing I've read.

The beautiful meshing of things together
Though some would but call it fate,
Like the sudden cry of a lone bird calling—
The quick answer of his mate.

A day in the fall when the breeze is blowing
The acorns come thudding down
And a look o'er the meadow where green was growing
Finds patches now turned to brown.

Or trees in the winter when leaves have fallen
Their limbs looking stark and bare,
We look away for a moment not watching—
A blanket of snow is there!

Oh, how can we live in the world not seeing
The beauty of earth we've trod?
Each "thing of beauty *is* a joy forever,"
And comes from the hand of God.

The doctor looked at me with compassion. He took my hands in his, as though to cushion the shock of his words.

"I am *so* sorry. It is what we feared most," he said of my husband. "Dick has cerebral atrophy (Alzheimer's disease) and it will get worse. It is not treatable and always fatal, though we cannot tell how long he will live. So far, there is no known cause or cure."

He stood as though reluctant to leave. I scarcely noticed as I watched them roll Dick past on his way to the recovery room. They had informed me that he would be monitored for a short while before being returned to his room.

After the doctor left, I stayed on in the waiting room. My heart was pounding and my body tense. I closed my eyes as I whispered, "Oh, God, no! Please, Lord, anything but this!"

It was difficult to realize that such a sentence had just been pronounced upon my Dick. He had always been so strong. I thought of how, at every routine physical, the doctors would laugh and say, "Get out of here, Dick Atkins, you're disgustingly healthy!"

His energy, his health, and his utter zest for living were such a part of him. His eyes literally danced most of the time.

I remembered the first time I ever saw him. In between teaching assignments, I had approached a Chrysler dealership with an innovative idea for a daily radio show. They bought it and Dick was assigned, as a newspaper photographer, to take my picture. I would be billed as "The Valiant Lady."

He came on schedule—a well-built man of average height, sleeves rolled to just below his elbows, a small hat pushed back on his head, and about the largest camera I had ever seen slung over his shoulder. And there was his smile. It was one that I could never describe, but shall never forget.

I remembered, too, the first thing he said that showed me how different he was from most men. Sometime later, but still early in our acquaintance, he confided, "I can't think of anything more wonderful than to be married to someone you could pray with!"

My heart responded warmly to these words. I had loved God almost all my life, and through the years, He had become increasingly real to me.

My friends had often asked, "What are you waiting for, perfection?" My answer was always the same. "Of course not, I'm not perfect." I never revealed the deep desire I had to share my life with someone who loved God as I did. But I always knew that without that, I was better off alone.

Up to that point, I had spent most of my adult life teaching and doing mission work in areas as far apart as Florida, Colorado, Arizona, California and Hawaii. I had worked among all kinds of people—Caucasians, Blacks, Navajo Indians, Hispanics, and Hawaiians.

From the time of our first meeting, Dick started asking me out. Though there was an instant rapport between us, I was reluctant. For by then my heart was turned in another direction. I had entered an Episcopal convent a few years before, but had to leave due to illness.

The spring Dick and I met, I had made plans to visit a number of convents again, to decide once and for all whether that was the life I wanted, or that God wanted for me.

Even though Dick seemed disappointed to learn that I would be gone most of the summer, he was understanding. He actually told me that if I decided to go, he would help me in any way he could— even drive me there. He asked me at least to drop him a card now and then, while I was away. I didn't.

Upon my return he was there, as considerate as ever. He said he would not try to influence me one way or the other, but would like for us to go out to dinner now and then.

Since I was still trying to arrive at a decision, I felt it best not to get involved. A very good friend chided me, however, saying, "You don't have to *marry* the man, you know. But since you are both alone, what's the harm in going out to dinner once in a while?"

Dick always chuckled afterwards remembering how I tried to make my position clear at our very first dinner together. "Dick," I said as soon as the waiter had taken our order, "I have to get one thing straight with you. If you want to go out occasionally, on a friendly basis, because you're alone and I'm alone, that's fine. But

I must tell you that I have no intention of getting serious with you!"

He smiled and said, "That's O.K. with me. Whatever you say."

Only a short time after that, I became ill again. While not too serious, it brought me to the reluctant acknowledgment that I did not have the physical stamina for the demanding life of a Religious. In addition, most entered younger than I. That dream died hard, for it had long been in my heart.

I said nothing to Dick about it, but almost as though he could read my thoughts, in a very short time he asked me to marry him. We had known each other only a few months, and it was three or four weeks since our first dinner together, but he seemed so sure. I wasn't. He was willing to wait, so we kept on seeing each other. I was struck often by his gentle manner and kindness.

Though it might seem a small thing, I shall never forget one incident so characteristic of him. We had been to the beach, and on our way home stopped at the grocery for a few things I needed. As we neared the check-out counter, Dick got out his wallet.

"No, Dick! These are mine. I'll pay for them!"

Dick turned to me quickly, his brown eyes shining with a special softness. "But, Marguerite, have you forgotten? I'm the guy who wants to buy your groceries for the rest of your life!"

After taking what seemed to both of us a very long month to seek guidance from God and spiritual counsel, I found my answer.

We were sitting at a desk littered with snapshots when I told Dick I would marry him. His face shone with joy as he cried, "Oh, Sweetheart, you'll never be sorry!" We both laughed when he added, "I'm going to make it my vocation in life to make you smile more. You're too serious!"

And how he did just that! His sense of humor was so contagious and his clowning so comical that I found myself laughing more often and more freely than at any time in my life. Whenever mention was made by anyone of the shortness of time between that first dinner and our marriage, his answer was a teasing one. "Well, I wasn't a fisherman for nothing! I knew how to give her plenty of line, and then, just reel her in very gently!"

Though we spent some time in California right after our marriage, we decided to live in Florida—my home state. Dick's parents had retired there from Ohio, and besides that, I had an invalid sister who was a patient in a nursing home, and longed to have us close by.

My parents and three brothers had died—the third during the time Dick and I were in California.

It wasn't long until we purchased and moved into our new house in Fort Myers, Florida. Those first months were filled with joy as we worked together to turn that house into a home. We were also busy at jobs we liked. Dick was with a small newspaper a few miles away, and I was teaching at a nearby elementary school.

Dick had lived in several states including Ohio, New York and Oregon. He had been a Physical Education major in college and had worked at a number of things. His favorite was as a Physical Therapist, for which he had received training in Chicago. But in Florida, he learned that he would have to go to school much longer than he wished in order to get a state license. He opted instead for newspaper work, at which he was also quite experienced.

As time passed, I learned how numerous and varied Dick's interests were. Mine had always run toward glee clubs, choirs, and drama—as participant and director—and Christian Education—as teacher, writer and public speaker. I loved children and had managed to sandwich in a bit of camp directing along the way.

Dick was an avid "rock-hound" and fossil collector. He liked sharing this knowledge with the science classes at my school. It was not at all unusual to have some bright-eyed fifth grader ring our door bell, ask for him and say, "Look, Mr. Atkins! Look what *I* found!" He also shared this interest with various garden clubs, who invited him to give talks and exhibit his collection.

He enjoyed fishing and often took me out in his boat, preferring to row rather than use the motor.

His enthusiasm for bird watching was contagious and we were soon signed up as members of the Audubon Club. He was never happier than on our Audubon outings—whether by river boat or sloshing through the swamps in high-top boots. He counted his binoculars among his most prized possessions.

Dick quickly became involved with the local Boy Scouts—a lifelong interest with him. He had been in scouting since he was twelve years old, except for the two years he spent with the Navy in North Africa. He had served in many capacities, but being an expert swimmer, he was particularly helpful to boys trying to pass their life-saving tests, or their swimming requirements for Eagle.

I soon learned that he had a deep and special love for St. Francis of Assissi, the patron saint of birds and animals. I sometimes teasingly called him "Nature Boy," but inwardly realized how much he exemplified the love and the joy of the great saint.

There seemed no end to all the things Dick enjoyed. At home he loved to cook, and often did. While in the kitchen, he was fond of striking a pose as he declared in an exaggerated tone: "In this house we don't need a dishwasher. We've got one—me!" In his *spare* time he liked to whittle, and we both liked to read.

In the evening, we loved to turn off all the lights, roll up the blinds on three sides of our paneled "Florida room" and watch the sky. Sometimes we listened to our favorite stereo records playing softly in the background. But more often we would just sit silently in the darkness, drinking in the quiet beauty of the night. Occasionally Dick would show me things about the stars that I had never seen or known.

We shared many activities and interests, but by far our deepest bond was our mutual love for God. We were both active at St. Luke's Church. I was chairman of Christian Education and Devotional Life for the women. Dick led a Scout troop, and was in charge of the eight o'clock ushers. Our times of prayer at home brought us closer to each other and to our Lord.

The heartsease that we felt was made up of a deeper understanding than I had dreamed possible. Oh, how I loved him! With trembling heart, many times over, I thanked God for Dick's love— and for *His* in giving us to each other.

Two

*First
Shadows*

Winged Gift

I wonder why the birds seem never sad
  Why they can sing
  How they can sing
  All the day long
And sing as cheerfully throughout the night.

Is there no time at all when joy runs cold
  When they are dry
  Indifferent
  Devoid of love . . .
To them is sadness utterly unknown?

When question I the remedy for pain
  How soothe the wounds
  Of sorrow deep
  I hear their call—
Their incessant cry—"Look up! Look up! Look up!"

But God's to know the fount from which it comes . . .
  For they are His gift
  Bright winged gift
  Created to sing
And lift sad mortals to His heart of love!

The first shadows fell upon our lives in 1969—seven years after we were married. At first they were so faint as to be almost unrecognizable. But by the end of the year they could no longer be ignored.

Those first seven years had been full and happy—ideally so. At times I wondered at having a husband who was so kind and loving—so fine and fine-looking.

It was not unusual, when we were with a group, to have one of our female friends ask me, in his presence, "Where did you ever find a handsome man like that?"

Dick never gave me time to answer. He would always jump in and say, "She didn't find me, I found her!" What wife wouldn't feel ten feet tall at such words from the one she loved?

In private as well as in public, Dick showered small kindnesses upon me. Of course he was kind to everyone, children and adults alike. But there were always those little extra touches of consideration for me, which showed how much he cared—and I loved it!

I particularly loved the way he had of remembering me with gifts and thoughtful cards. He was overly generous in this respect—especially at Christmas, Valentine's Day, Easter, my birthday and on our anniversary. The latter three fell close together, in the springtime. At whichever one came last, he delighted in teasing me by saying, "Well, Sweetie, you know how it is around our house. It's feast or famine. You've had your feast, now it's going to be famine for you until Christmas!" We always shared a good laugh over this.

It was not surprising, then, that Dick's failure to remember me on Valentine's Day that year cast the first very faint shadow. When I gave him his card and gift, he seemed genuinely sorry that he had forgotten. I rationalized that everyone forgets sometime.

But when he forgot the other special spring days as well—*all* of them—I was both hurt and puzzled. Was he beginning to love me less? I wondered.

Throughout the summer, things went along pretty much as usual. One could not stay at outs with Dick for very long—he was so dear and loving. Just to be with him was to be caught up in his joy of living.

One fall evening, when dinner was over and the dishes out of the way, I was sitting comfortably in a recliner out in the Florida room (so called in our part of the country because of its expanse of windows and comfortable decor). The spectacular beauty of the slowly fading sunset was more than relaxing. It gave me a feeling of deep contentment.

Dick was off in the house someplace. Through the window, I saw him walk into the kitchen and open a cupboard door. He quickly closed it. Then he opened and closed another—and yet another.

"What are you looking for, Honey?"

"Oh, just a glass to get a drink of water," he answered. "Never mind, I found it."

Now this would hardly have seemed significant to anyone else, but I suddenly felt uneasy. Why? I wondered. The glasses had been in the same place during all the years we had lived there.

The rest of the evening was uneventful. It was one of those looking at the sky, listening to music kind. Dick acted so naturally that I wondered if I had been too quick to worry. How *could* anything be wrong?

By bedtime, I had convinced myself that it was merely my overactive imagination. But that night I lay awake longer than usual, while my husband slept peacefully beside me. I did not know it then, but the shadows had only begun to fall.

The next couple of days were busy ones for both of us. I usually arose at six o'clock sharp, since I had to be in my schoolroom by seven-thirty. Although Dick didn't have to be at his office until nine, he liked to get up in time for us to have a short prayer together before I left, and to see me off.

The third morning after the incident of the glass, I was almost ready to leave when he came quickly out to the utility room next to the carport, where we often said our goodbyes. "Sweetheart," he asked hurriedly, "is tonight my Scout night?"

"No, that's tomorrow night."

"Oh, of course, that's right."

As we embraced, we bowed our heads and he said a short prayer for me. Then he looked up with a mischievous grin and winked. "I

25

sure do love you, Teacher," he said.

"You too," I laughed, "now close those eyes so I can pray for you."

I liked to say the same prayer for him each morning. (More leisurely prayers and reading from the Bible and some spiritual book were saved for later in the day, when we had more time.) With our eyes closed and with hands and foreheads touching, I prayed for him: "Oh, God, bless this Thy servant, Richard. Keep him in safety and protection. Give him health of body, peace of mind and joy of heart. And make him a blessing to others. Amen."

A quick kiss and a "Bye, Honey!" saw me out the door, hurrying to my car. This time Dick followed me. "Sweetie, wait! I meant to ask you something. Is tonight Scout night?"

My heart skipped a beat. I hesitated for a moment. "Dick, you just asked me that a little while ago, and I told you it's tomorrow night. Don't you remember?"

"Oh," he said, "guess you're right."

As I drove away, I carried with me a picture of the puzzled look on his face. The little knot of worry was back. Only this time, it was larger. I felt more troubled than at any time for years.

The uneasy feeling lingered. All during the day, quick prayers kept winging their way upward. "Oh, God, show me what is wrong." (I knew something had to be.) "Dear Lord, please help him . . . and me. Please be with us."

Sometime in the afternoon, a particular verse of Scripture came to me: "Lo, I am with you alway, even unto the end of the world." (Matt. 28:20) I kept thinking about it, for the words brought me a measure of solace.

Even so, I found that for the first time since we were married, I had mixed feelings about going home. I longed for the comfort of Dick's arms around me, but knew that this time I could not tell him why.

Though Dick's question about the scout meeting was the first one he repeated, it was not to be his last. As he came more often to ask me a question which I had answered thirty minutes—or even five minutes—before, I tried to be patient. But sometimes, especially at the end of a trying day, I was apt to say, "Dick, I just *told* you that. Didn't you listen?"

It was quite a shock one evening when he got very upset over this and snapped, "Don't treat me like one of your school children!" With that, he stormed out the front door, slamming it behind him, and didn't return for several hours. When he did come home, he went straight to bed, refusing to talk.

From the beginning, Dick and I had been especially close. We never argued and quarreled like some couples—seldom even disagreed. But these episodes began to flare up so suddenly, that the damage would be done before I realized it.

To see him rush out of the house like that, in the middle of an otherwise companionable time (usually in the evening) was heartbreaking. I could only wait the hour—or two—or three—until he finally came home and quietly crawled into bed.

Such a rift between us was unthinkable, so I began to try to talk with him. I would tell him how much I loved and missed him, and of my regret at having upset him. I tried, in every way possible, to draw him out of the silence that seemed to have him locked in.

The most effective approach, I soon found, was to kneel beside him and pray the St. Francis prayer. He loved that prayer so much that it had come to have a special significance for us both.

So, with my arm around him and my face touching his, I would pray softly:

O Lord, make us instruments of Your peace!

> Where there is hatred, let us sow love;
> Where there is injury, pardon;
> Where there is doubt, faith;
> Where there is despair, hope;
> Where there is darkness, light; and
> Where there is sadness, joy.

O Divine Master, grant that we may not so much seek to be consoled, as to console;

> To be understood, as to understand;
> To be loved, as to love;
> For, it is in giving, that we receive;
> It is in pardoning, that we are pardoned; and
> It is dying, that we are born to eternal life.

Dick seemed unable, at such a time, to join in as he ordinarily would. I could feel the tension drain out of him, however, as I neared the end. He would press my hand when I kissed him goodnight. The following morning, except for being somewhat subdued, he was usually his same sweet self.

Though I did not understand why he asked the same questions

repeatedly, I soon learned with what care I must answer them.

As the weeks passed, other things happened that puzzled me. One in particular, I remember, showed a sudden change of attitude on his part, concerning necessary household errands. From the beginning, he had insisted on doing them. I had tried to talk him out of it, saying, "Honey, I get home much earlier than you."

"But it's easier for me," he would say, "I'm in and out of my car all day long. I cover a lot of territory while you're confined to your schoolroom." Then he would joke, "You'd better 'let George do it'!" Thus the pattern of his doing the greater part of our errands was established.

His reaction, then, on one morning when I asked him to pick up something we needed came as a complete surprise: "Marguerite, you're just making nothing but an errand boy out of me!" His tone of voice was totally unlike him.

Startled, but not wanting to show it, I quickly said, "Never mind. If you're going to be too busy today, I'll get it after school. It's all right." I decided then not to ask him to do any more errands.

As the weeks turned into months, other changes brought a growing sense of apprehension. At times I could see how confused he became over things which he had always done quickly and with ease.

One evening stands out quite vividly. I was reading in the Florida room, where we spent most of our leisure time, when it suddenly dawned on me that I hadn't seen Dick in more than an hour. I went to find out what he was doing.

He was at the desk in the living room, pen in hand, hunched over his checkbook. (We had two checking accounts, which we both used. He had always kept track of one and I, the other.) I saw at once his frown of worry. "Hi, I miss you. Are you almost finished?" I said. His troubled look, as he turned to me, seemed all out of proportion to what he was doing.

"Oh, guess I'm just having a little bit of trouble with this," he sighed. "Want to take a look?"

With the first glance, I was stunned. His figures made no sense at all. Intuitively, I knew I must not let on.

"Sweetheart," I managed casually, "You've worked long enough. Come on, let's turn off the lights, and you tell me about the stars, O.K.?"

"But . . ."

"No buts about it. I'll be home much earlier than you tomorrow. I'll look over it then. I promise!" He smiled in obvious relief.

The next afternoon he seemed to have forgotten all about it. It was not hard at all, several days later, to convince him that there was really little point in our having two checking accounts. He readily agreed that we should combine them. From then on, I took care of all our financial matters. He never seemed to notice.

As the year passed, my apprehension continued to grow. What is happening to us? I wondered over and over. I prayed often and fervently during those painful and perplexing months—mostly prayers of distress and supplication.

"Oh, Blessed God, pour into my heart a deeper love for You, and for Dick. Help me to help him. Bestow upon me all wisdom, to see and to follow Your will."

I felt sure that our Lord would bring this to pass in His own time and way. But, at the moment, I saw only the deepening shadows. The answer to the 'what' and the 'why' of it all eluded me.

Three

Mounting Concern

The Brimming Cup

I cannot see nor can I know the things Thou holdest
Out in love in nail-pierced hands.
   The hands are Thine
      And Thou art love
   Thus I receive
      With love not mine
The cup that's brimming with Thy love divine. Oh, grant me
Grace to drink it, nor repine.

More and more, our life together became one of ups and downs. Almost every time something happened that caused me to worry, Dick would do something so in character that I wondered why I did. At times I would feel sure that something was wrong with him, only to have his actions belie the thought. It was a bit like being on a roller coaster, not knowing how to get off.

I began to notice that he seemed less positive about his work. He was an advertising salesman and layout artist for his paper, and had always been quite proficient at it. Now, I sensed that while he was beginning to worry about his accounts, he was spending less time on them.

He always seemed to find time for any Boy Scout who needed his help. But then scouting was high on his list of priorities. As a matter of fact, it hadn't been too long since he was presented with the coveted Wood Badge Award—the first man in Lee County to receive it. That took a great deal of skill as well as hard work. Yet, now he depended on me to help him remember not only the day when his troop met, but what he had told me were his plans for the next meeting.

The same was true about church. For some years he had been responsible for seeing that ushers were on hand each Sunday morning for the eight o'clock service. Now, he either forgot to call them, or when he did, was sometimes unsure of what to say. This caused me deep concern.

Dick continued to be very helpful around the house. He cautioned me many times not to touch the vacuum, as that was his job. As always, he liked to help me by washing the dishes. And on the few occasions when I was frustrated at having scorched a pan, he would say, "Don't worry about it. I'll clean it for you." He did, and it was usually shinier than brand new when he finished.

As the months dragged on into still another year, I continued to observe him closely. It was then that I began to detect a faint pattern in Dick's actions. He seemed comfortable in the things we did together, and relaxed in those that were recreational. But I sensed that he was growing less able to stand pressure of any kind, and that he was finding it increasingly difficult to deal with details. This could explain his reluctance to do errands, and his confusion about his job.

The changes in my beloved husband were becoming more apparent all the time. But I simply could not understand why. I kept searching for an answer.

I knew that Dick's father had grown more and more forgetful and confused in late years. He was then being cared for in a local nursing home, where he was said to be suffering from hardening of the arteries. I kept wondering if that was Dick's trouble. But Dad is close to eighty, I kept telling myself, and Dick is only in his mid–fifties—and looks and acts much younger!

In spite of my inner arguments, the question persisted: Could that be it? I had to find out. Knowing that I might be grasping at a very weak straw, I decided to try and get him to a doctor.

More time went by, before I could finally get up the courage to broach the subject. When I did, his response did not surprise me. He denied, vehemently, that anything was wrong with him. "Honey, you know how every doctor that I've ever seen has said I'm 'disgustingly healthy,' and I feel fine. The doctor would just laugh at me!"

Now, I am no different from any other wife who loves and knows she is loved in return. "Then do it for me, Dick, please!"

He never could resist when I put it like that. "Aw . . ." He hesitated for a moment. "Oh, all right. I guess I'll do it for you. But I'm sure the doctor won't find anything."

The next morning I made the appointment, but my request either to go in with him, or at least to talk with the doctor by telephone, was denied. "Mr. Atkins is perfectly capable of telling the doctor whatever he needs to know," the secretary told me over the phone. I did not feel at all sure that was true but, nevertheless, had to accept it.

On the appointed day I drove to the office with him, and waited. For me, the time he spent with the doctor seemed endless. Once we were in the car, I questioned him. "What did he say, Honey?"

"He said there's nothing wrong with me."

"What did you tell him, Dick? Did you explain anything at all?"

"Well, I told him my wife thought I might be getting hardening of the arteries, because I forget sometimes."

"And?"

"He just checked me over and said I was O.K."

"Are you sure that's *all* he said?" I was feeling very anxious and frustrated.

Dick thought hard for a moment before he answered. "Well, he said several things, but I can't remember them all . . . Oh, yes! He did say my arteries are like those of a young man, and I only need to concentrate more!"

Dick was so delighted that it had turned out so well that I didn't have the heart to tell him how I felt. We rode in silence for several minutes. Then he turned to me and said, "You know something? You don't act glad at all. What's the matter? Did you *want* him to find something wrong with me?"

I patted his arm. "Darling, you know me better than that."

After our evening meal, Dick decided to fish for a while in the Orange River, across the street. This gave me some time alone, to think. Regardless of what the doctor had said, *I didn't believe him.* My concern, which had mounted slowly over the past few years, but more rapidly during past weeks and days, was now intensified. I had a very strong inner feeling that this was no time to stop—that something had to be done!

"O God, guide me," I prayed that evening. "Please show me what to do." In His mercy, He did. While Dick was still fishing across the way, the answer came. I would call Father Haynes, our parish priest, the very next day. I had to talk with someone, and knew that he cared about us both.

That night I slept a bit more easily.

The next morning, I left my classroom long enough to call Father Haynes. He said he would be in his office at four o'clock.

After we were seated that afternoon with the door closed, I had a good feeling about being there. Father Haynes was a big man with an even bigger heart. His manner was warm and inviting as he asked me to tell him what was on my mind. (I had kept him informed of some of the changes in Dick, and knew he shared my concern.)

Briefly I brought him up to date, telling him in particular about Dick's visit to the doctor. I told him of my disappointment that he had been so casual about it and had told Dick that nothing was wrong.

"There *is* something wrong, Father Haynes—I know it! I live with him and he is not the same man he used to be."

Father Haynes nodded. "Marguerite, I agree that Dick is not like he used to be. I've noticed that when he offers to help out down here at the church, he often fails to show up. That's not at all like Dick. So the question is not *whether* something is wrong, but how we can go about finding out what. Do you have any ideas at all?"

I told him that even before I made the appointment with the local doctor, I'd wanted Dick to see the head of Neurology at Shands Teaching Hospital at the University of Florida, in Gainesville. I had met Dr. Greer a year or so earlier and was impressed with his expertise and warmth. It had seemed easier to talk Dick into seeing a doctor near home, however, so I'd settled on that.

"I'd like the best in the world to have him go to Shands, Father. They are well known for their diagnostic work. But now, I'm afraid Dick won't go anywhere else—not even to please me."

Father Haynes sat for a moment, thinking. I knew that look, so I waited. He suddenly leaned toward me; his eyes were full of compassion. "Would you like for me to see if I can get him to go?"

"Oh Father, do you think you could?"

"Well, I can certainly give it a try. H'mm . . . Tomorrow's Saturday," he mused. "I'll call him early, before he gets busy with something else." And so it was arranged.

The next morning the telephone rang around nine. Dick answered. I heard him say: "Hi, Father . . . No, I'm not busy . . . Sure, I'll be glad to come . . . Of course, Father. I'll come right away."

With a questioning look, he turned to me. "That was Father Haynes—he said he wanted to see me. Wonder what he wants to see me about? Do you suppose he wants me to start another Scout troop or something?"

"Well, old Buddy, the only way to find out is to go down and see," I teased. "So you'd better get going!"

I stayed close to the phone during the next hour or more. Sure enough, Father Haynes called so that we could talk before Dick got home.

"What happened, Father?"

"It couldn't have gone better," he began. "I decided not to beat around the bush. So as soon as he was settled I came right to the point. 'Marguerite is very worried about you, Dick, and wants you to go up to Shands Hospital in Gainesville, to see a neurologist. Will you go?' I think he was so surprised, that he agreed on the spot.

I don't believe you'll have any trouble about it."

I felt so relieved, that my only reply was "Thanks, Father."

He was right. Dick offered no objections. The appointment was made for a week from the following Tuesday. I thought I sensed not only a willingness to go on Dick's part, but an indefinable touch of relief as well.

That afternoon, while shopping in one of our large department stores, I ran into Dick's employer—the publisher of his paper. I was glad, for I had planned to call her. Seeing her was much better.

I explained about Dick's appointment at Shands—why we were going and the uncertainty of how long he would need to be away. Her response was both warm and supportive.

"Marguerite, I'm so relieved that he is going!" she said. "We've thought for a long while that something was different about Dick. It has been much more noticeable these past few months."

"Jo, why didn't you say something to me?" I questioned.

"We were so unsure about it, Marguerite, and we didn't know whether you had noticed or not. We are all so fond of Dick, and we didn't want to hurt him—or you, either, for that matter."

We talked on for a few minutes and she urged me to take all the time we needed. As we parted she said, "Please keep us posted. If the doctor decides to keep him, call us collect. Please feel free to call us collect *anytime*."

The night before Dick and I were to leave, I waited until he was asleep and put two small bags, which I had packed for us, into the trunk of the car. I had also a typed list of all the changes I had seen in him in the past two or three years. Though his appointment was only as an outpatient, I meant to be prepared for anything, and hoped that the doctor would have him admitted.

I didn't go to bed for a long while. The quiet hours gave me needed time to think and to pray. This was a big step, but the right one, I felt certain. No matter what happened, we could find out *something*. Hopefully, we—or at least I—would no longer be fumbling in the dark.

"O God, I love him so much. But I know that You love him even more. Help me to give him into Your hands," I prayed. "He loves You, Lord, and I love You. Strenghten us both to rest in Your love. Whatever the outcome of this trip, please keep us in Your will and in Your spirit. Above all, grant us Your peace."

With the "Amen" still in my heart, I walked toward our bedroom. Slipping in noiselessly beside Dick, his dear face was clearly visible in the moonlight. I reached out and touched it gently, and was struck anew by the almost childlike quality it reflected—by his look of utter peace.

As I settled down for sleep, the loveliness of the night sounds could be heard: a lone owl, the crickets, and the sweet but mournful cry of the whippoorwills in the distance. For their accompaniment, a soft breeze was brushing a palm frond gently across our window.

Into my mind came the words: "Peace I leave with you, my peace I give unto you. Let not your heart be troubled, neither let it be afraid." (John 14:27) God's peace filled my heart. His love enveloped us both. My deep desire, at that moment, was not to be afraid. I wanted to trust Him, no matter what might lie ahead.

Somehow, that night, I knew that God would give me—would continue to give me—the trust that I needed. "Yes, Lord," I whispered as I gave Dick a light kiss. "Yes, Lord," I murmured over and over, until I finally fell asleep.

Four

The Appointment

Clouds

Little puffs of eyelet clouds
Nestled o'er the green,
Farther out white islands, in
Assorted shapes are seen.

Blazing in brief resplendence
From the sun, and then
Back to softer quietness
Of white on blue again.

Looking toward the horizon,
A discerning eye
Finds that the islands (or the clouds?)
Melt into the sky.

Could it be, our troubles—
Our little bits of pain—
Melt into Thy heavenly love
Where there they may remain?

O Lord of all Creation,
Let us rest in Thee, we pray,
As effortlessly as the clouds
Float in the sky today.

The next morning, after a quick breakfast, we got off early. It was about a four or five hour drive to Gainesville. (There was no Interstate then.) The early start would get us there in plenty of time to locate the hospital, have lunch, and keep the appointment at two-thirty.

Dick wasn't very talkative the first hour, though usually he was happy and carefree when we were on a trip. He had insisted on driving, and I could not think of a good enough reason to object. Inwardly, I thought his driving was becoming somewhat erratic— but I wasn't sure.

We drove in silence for quite some time before I said, "A penny for your thoughts, Honey."

"Oh, I was just thinking how different this trip is from all the others we've taken. They were fun!"

"We have had some good times together, haven't we?" I said, knowing it was better to get his thoughts on something pleasant than have him dwelling on what lay ahead. "Remember our trip to Jamaica?"

It took only a few minutes of reminiscing to bring him back to his usual cheerful self. We talked for a while about our two weeks in Jamaica. We had gone there because of our interest in our then "Companion Diocese."

Though we had made reservations for each place we intended to visit, we soon found our plans changed by three island families. They were all Anglican—two of them headed by priests. Due to their thoughtfullness and their warm hospitality, we had found our experiences far different from those of the usual tourists. Jamaica had indeed been a high point for both of us.

As we continued on toward Gainesville, we remembered also,

our last trip to Ohio to visit Dick's daughter, Karen. Then, with eyes shining, he said, "You know what I enjoyed most of anything we've ever done?"

"I have an idea, but you tell me."

"Remember that time we stopped for a few days in Franklin, North Carolina? I spent most of my time out where people were sitting by those troughs, with the water and the mud coming down, trying to find gemstones. I found some pretty good ones, too. Remember?"

I remembered, all right. But I simply could not understand how he remembered things so clearly from years past, but seemed unable to recall things more recent.

Time went faster now, with Dick in a more cheerful frame of mind. We talked and sang the miles away. Before long we were on the outskirts of Gainesville. After stopping for lunch, we found the hospital with little trouble. Soon we were in the waiting room, with time to spare.

I managed to slip my typewritten notes to the nurse at the desk, without Dick knowing. She promised that the doctor would read them before Dick was called.

He did better than that—he asked me to come in first. We discussed my observations briefly, before he asked me to call my husband. I don't know how long Dick spent with him—it no doubt seemed longer than it really was. I only know that my hands were icy as I waited for him. The question uppermost in my mind was, I wonder what he will find? I felt sure that he would find something. I hoped that it would not be too bad, but feared, at the same time, what he might say. In my heart the prayers were constant.

At last Dick appeared, with a nurse walking beside him. His face gave me no clue as to what had happened. "Mrs. Atkins," she said, "the doctor would like to speak with you again. Mr. Atkins, you can wait right here—it won't be long." She spoke with kindness to us both.

I felt, as I walked again toward the doctor's office, that my heart was being squeezed—*hard*. It was difficult to breathe. "Oh, God, help us, be with us," I prayed silently.

"Mrs. Atkins," he began after we were seated. "You are right. I'm afraid there *is* something wrong with your husband. I asked him a number of questions and tried to get him to follow several specific instructions. He tried, but I could see that he was totally confused."

"Oh, Doctor, these are the kinds of things that have had me so worried. What is it? What's causing it? Can anything be done?"

"Mrs. Atkins, I know you are concerned. There are several things that can cause forgetfulness and confusion. Some are simple to correct—most of them we can help. Others, however, are more difficult, and one or two are untreatable. The first thing we need to do is to run some tests. I'd like to have him admitted to the hospital. Do you think he will agree?"

"I was hoping you would say that, and I came prepared. Let me go and talk with him."

"Dear God," I prayed as I walked hurriedly toward Dick, "please let him say 'yes' if that is Your will. Oh, please help him."

I was surprised at the ease with which Dick agreed. (God was answering my prayer.) "Well, we've come this far," he said, "I guess we might as well go all the way."

I hugged him as I whispered, "Darling, I love you." We walked back to the Neurology desk, hand in hand.

The nurse gave me his room number and then suggested that I look up the social worker on the first floor, who would help me find a place to stay. She paused long enough to tell me that he would be alone, for the time being, in a semi-private room and that I was free to see him at any time.

My heart was tight as she led him away. My face must have mirrored my feelings, for Dick had taken only a few steps when he turned to me and smiled. "Don't worry, Sweetie. It's all right. I'll be waiting for you!"

It took quite a while to get the necessary information about the home where I would be staying, to find it and then to make arrangements with the landlord. Once there, I unpacked my bag quickly, then I returned to the hospital and went straight to Dick's room.

He was half sitting on his bed when I arrived. His eyes showed his joy at seeing me. "Oh, my little Dove," he said as he drew me close. (That was one of his two most endearing names for me). I ran my hands through his black, wavy hair as he held me for a moment.

"I can't believe this," he laughed as he leaned back and propped his elbow against the pillow. "I can't believe it—me, here in this hospital—when I don't even feel sick!"

For all his jesting, he finally admitted that evening—for the very first time—that he had been more concerned than he had wanted me to know. "I hope they can help me," he said. "At the rate I'm forgetting everything, I won't be able to hold a job for another two years!"

With this opening, I knew we could talk. And talk we did, on a level and in a manner that we had not done for almost three long and perplexing years. My heart was thankful for that.

I was even more thankful to hear him speak freely again, of his feelings about God. "He knows we love Him. And we know He loves us. We don't need to worry. Whatever happens, we will still be in His hands. Oh, my sweetheart," he said as his eyes looked tenderly into mine, "He'll watch over us. We just have to trust Him."

I agreed, trying to hold back the tears. My love for Dick had never been greater. From my heart went a quick prayer of thanksgiving for the spiritual oneness we shared.

Not until I was safely in bed that night could I let the tears come. They must have been building for a very long time and it was good to get them out. Afterward, I was surprised at the strange and unexpected feeling of release—as though I had been cleansed.

This was the first time in years that Dick and I had been separated. I missed him, but was convinced, beyond any doubt, that he was in good hands—*God's.*

Five

Shands:
Days of
Waiting

The Mantle of Thy Love

Oh, help me, Lord, to drink life's bitter potion,
My share of sorrow clasp unto my breast;
Knowing Thy love surrounds, upholds and keeps me
Will enable me to come to Thee and rest.

Let the mantle of Thy love fall upon me,
Tender whisper of Thy love fall on my heart;
Then when sorrow comes, threatening to destroy me,
I can know, O Lord, I share Thy grief, in part.

When I left Dick that first evening in the hospital, I had no idea what to expect. I didn't know what kind of tests would be given to him, nor how they would go about trying to pinpoint the trouble. But when I reached his room the next morning, it was apparent they had already begun. His bed was freshly made and Dick was not there. The nurse told me that the orderly had come for him early, as the Neurology staff was "anxious to get started."

During the next few days it seemed that he was out of his room more than he was in it. I spent much of my time waiting for him, as I wandered around from one part of the hospital to the other.

Dick couldn't tell me much about the tests he was taking, for most of them he didn't understand. He seemed very interested, however, in the psychological test that was administered and was able to tell me a little about that. (It had been explained to me earlier that it was necessary to "cover all the bases.")

After several days, one of the young interns was directed to bring me up to date on what was going on. He found me in the hospital cafeteria one morning and we talked over breakfast. He tried to explain some of the procedures, and why they were necessary. Even with his explanation, there were many things I did not understand, and the few that I did have now become a bit hazy, due to the lapse of time.

I do remember his telling me that the psychological test didn't show anything unusual—which indicated that Dick's trouble was probably organic. He spoke of another test that had involved a tiny atomic particle which had been monitored carefully as it travelled up the spinal column and through the brain. I don't recall the specific purpose of that one, but it had proved negative. Another test involved checking the thyroid. I had been told in my first consultation that confusion and forgetfulness could sometimes be caused by something as simple as an "off-kilter thyroid." That, too, had proved negative.

The young doctor could tell that I did not follow all he was saying. He also observed, I am sure, that I was feeling the strain and had hardly touched my food. On an impulse, he reached out and covered my hand with his. His eyes were warm and understanding as he said, "Mrs. Atkins, try not to worry. We're doing all that we can for him. I'm sure we'll be able to find the problem." Then, as he stood up, he added, smiling, "You know, that's some husband of yours. We're all amazed at his cheerfulness and courage!"

After he left, I dropped my head into my hands and prayed: "Oh, God, thank You. Thank You for all these kind doctors—please help them to find out what's wrong." Then, to Dick, as though my thoughts could travel to him, "Oh, Honey, I love you. I love you so much."

The tests went on. Saturday morning when I arrived I found Dick pacing up and down the hall outside his room. His eyes brightened as he hurried toward me, exclaiming, "Hi, there, am I glad to see *you*!" Then he told me that he had no tests scheduled for that day and only one on Sunday morning. At Shands, as at most hospitals, only the more urgent needs of the patients were looked after on the weekend.

"I don't mind the tests so much," Dick said as we entered his room. "But it's not going to be any fun being cooped up here for two whole days. I wish there was something we could do!"

I had not intended to tell him that it was my birthday. But seeing his restlessness, I decided to try and work something out that would lift his spirits.

"Honey, I want you to sit right here by the window and wait for me. I won't be gone long," I said.

"Where are you going?" he asked quickly. "What are you going to do?"

"You'll see. I'll be right back. I have an idea and it may just work. Keep your fingers crossed!"

I hurried to the nurses' station to see if it was O.K. for Dick to leave the floor. The nurse quickly wrote out a pass. She seemed glad to give it and said he could go anywhere in the hospital so long as he was not alone.

Dick's curiosity and interest showed on his face as I entered the room. "What is it?" he wanted to know. "I can tell you're up to something!"

"Well, Mr. Atkins," I teased, "your wife has just negotiated a pass for you. We can go anywhere in this hospital that your heart desires!"

His smile was back. "Well, lead on, Mrs. Atkins. I know you have something up your sleeve!"

On the elevator I mentioned that it was my birthday and that we were going to celebrate—making sure, of course, that he didn't blame himself for not remembering.

The gift shop—quite a nice one—was on the first floor. Dick was delighted that he could get something for me. He looked inside his wallet, which I had slipped into his bathrobe pocket, and with a laugh, instructed me in no uncertain terms to wait for him outside the door.

The kind saleswoman, who must have been accustomed to waiting upon patients who needed help, offered her assistance. I was glad, for with all the things to choose from, I knew that he might become confused.

When he came out, proudly carrying two beautifully wrapped packages, his eyes were shining. That was birthday present enough for me! This time he led *me* to the elevator saying that first we were going up to his room where I should open my gifts. After that, he announced, we were going to the cafeteria for a "bang-up" birthday dinner—his treat. And that's exactly what we did.

He really enjoyed that day and so did I. I still cherish the two gifts he chose for me: a set of aqua tulip bowls—dessert size—and a pair of small, white ceramic "kissing angels," which he said looked "just like us." I cherish even more the memory of that joyous day.

He held me a bit closer that evening as we said goodnight, and offered up a simple prayer of thanksgiving "for all our blessings."

Driving from the hospital to my room, I, too, lifted my heart in love and thanksgiving to God. Also, in my heart was what had become my constant plea—though perhaps not always articulated—that we might both continue to trust Him. I asked Him to be with Dick and to give him peace. I prayed for His strength to face whatever might lie ahead in the days to come.

Sunday was rather a leisurely day. Except for attending a nearby Episcopal Church service in the morning, while Dick was having his one scheduled test, I did very little. On Monday the usual hospital routine resumed with an accelerated round of tests for Dick.

When I reached his floor after lunch on Tuesday the nurse handed me a note from the same young doctor who had talked with me before. He asked me to meet him in the coffee shop downstairs before going into Dick's room. By that time I had learned that he was one of a team of seventeen doctors working on Dick's case. He had obviously been appointed their spokesman.

"I have been asked to talk with you again, Mrs. Atkins," he said as soon as we were seated. Then he told me that with all the tests that had been administered, they had not yet found the exact cause of Dick's trouble. "We believe that we are very close, however," he went on. "We know that there are only four things left that it could be: a brain tumor, which hopefully, could be helped by surgery; a blood clot, which can usually be dissolved; communicating hydrocephalus . . ."

"What is that?" I interrupted.

"Well," he paused as though trying to find a simple explanation. "The brain tissue usually floats rather freely on a sort of sea of liquid. Sometimes, for one reason or another, there is a blockage. That's what we call 'communicating hydrocephalus.' But these three conditions can almost always be treated successfully," he hastened to add.

"And the fourth?" I asked apprehensively.

His expression became grave. "Mrs. Atkins, the fourth one is cerebral atrophy, or the dying of the brain cells. Sometimes it's called 'Alzheimer's disease', after the doctor who first discovered that it was an organic brain disease—not merely the result of aging." He sensed my thoughts. "I have to tell you that this is the one condition that we don't know too much about. So far, medical scientists have not been able to find the cause. And until we do . . ." he shook his head, "there is nothing that can be done."

"How can you tell which of these my husband has?"

"To date, there is only one procedure which can give us an answer, and that's the pneumo-encephalogram."* He explained that Dick would be given an anesthetic and while strapped into a revolving chair, pictures of the brain would be taken from every angle. These would be much better than ordinary x-rays, and would tell, finally, what was causing Dick's trouble.

He paused, "There's just one thing, though. For this procedure to be performed, both you and Mr. Atkins will need to sign a consent form."

"Why? Is it dangerous?"

"Not necessarily," he answered. "It's hospital routine for any

*That was in 1972. Today the CAT SCAN is used.

49

patient who is given an anesthetic. But the risk in this case is minimal. I don't believe you should be too concerned about it.''

Before we parted, he told me that the doctor who was to supervise the procedure would come to Dick's room right after dinner to explain it to him, and to have us sign the form.

He came—right on schedule—and was most kind as he talked with Dick. It was evident to me, however, that he was stressing the procedure itself rather than going into any detail as to what they might find. When he finished, Dick seemed a bit tired and signed the form quickly, as though he just wanted to get it over with. I signed my name under his.

He was quiet after the doctor left and said—quite early for him—that he thought he had better get some sleep. "You too, Honey," he added with the ghost of a smile. Then he turned away from me and closed his eyes.

I stood uncertainly for a moment. Then I leaned over and kissed him on the cheek, and went out into the darkness to drive to my room, where I would spend a very restless night.

The next morning—Wednesday—Dick seemed his usual cheery self, laughing and teasing as we waited for what he termed the "big one." If he felt any apprehension, he didn't let on—not even when the orderlies came at one o'clock to roll him downstairs. He laughed and joked with them, but I felt his hand gripping mine tightly all the way down on the elevator and along the hall to the appointed room.

Since the door was left slightly ajar, I stood outside and watched as they strapped him into the chair, and administered the anesthetic.

When they realized that I was watching, one of the doctors came out and closed the door, suggesting very kindly that it would be better if I stayed in the waiting room. He walked with me, holding my arm, and saw me settled into a chair. I was glad for his support for my knees felt like rubber, my fast–beating pulse like hammers, and my hands were clammy.

As I sat there, unmoving, I faced the possibility, for the very first time since it had all begun three long years before, that Dick might never be himself again—that he might never get well. With this thought, my deep love for him became mixed with a sudden and overwhelming fear. It was so overpowering that I honestly don't remember whether I prayed or not. If so, it was most likely from my subconscious. Outwardly, I was conscious only of what was going on in that room, and what the consequences might be.

The time seemed endless. I had been told that the procedure

would take "only an hour or so" with a short time in the recovery room. They had thought he would be back in his room by three. A large clock, quietly ticking away on the wall, told me that Dick had already been in there much longer than that.

Just as my fear was beginning to turn to panic, the door opened and the doctor in charge came toward me. I searched his face for some sign that all was well. There was none.

It was then that he leaned over me, took my hands, and said with deep compassion, "Oh, Mrs. Atkins, I'm *so* sorry!"

The long hours that I waited beside my husband's empty bed for him to be brought back from the recovery room were filled with memories—a hazy kaleidoscope of thoughts and emotions. I left his room only long enough to call his mother, his employer, and the local priest, who had been so supportive during the past week. I decided all other calls could wait until we returned home.

Dick was finally wheeled in, at exactly seven o'clock and quickly transferred to his bed. After the nurse recorded his vital signs, we were left alone. He hardly moved as I sat beside him. His eyes were closed and only an occasional soft moan told me that he was not asleep. He spoke only twice, once when he murmured, "Oh, my head, my head," and once when he asked me to put a wet cloth over his eyes. This was the first time that I had ever seen Dick ill.

I do not know how long I stayed with him. The nurse came in after several hours and said, "Mrs. Atkins, don't you think you'd better go? You need some rest. He'll be all right. We'll take very good care of him. I promise!"

I do not remember driving back to my room. But I remember all too well the pain and the grief of that long, long night. I remember, also, the refrain from somewhere deep within me which kept repeating itself: "Lord have mercy. *Christ, have mercy.* Lord, have mercy."

This was interspersed occasionally, during those endless hours, by a sharper cry: "O God! . . . oh, *dear God!*"

Sometime in the quiet hours before daybreak, I finally fell asleep.

Six

Heading
Home

Night's Blanket

Red sun peeks through waving trees
The evening's soft with scented breeze
    And God is in His world.

Green leaves dance, fluttering, in their glee
And birds make merry melody
    As night's blanket is unfurled.

Sky's softer hues replace at last
The brilliant colors, fading fast,
    Their final rays all hurled.

While grasses nestle down to stay
Night creatures at the close of day
    Ready for sleep are curled.

As darkness softly settles down
In shades of grey and shades of brown
The quiet whisper of each sound
    Says: "God *is* in His world!"

I learned when I reached Dick's floor on Thursday morning that our ten long days at Shands were about over. Dick was out in the hall with several of his doctors. They really liked him and had come to say goodbye before hurrying to their respective duties.

As soon as I arrived, the doctor who had administered the test the day before informed us that Dick could be dismissed. "Now that the tests are completed," he said, turning toward him, "you don't have to stay any longer."

Forestalling questions, he went on. "We found that you have a memory problem, Mr. Atkins, and you will need to learn to live with it. The best way to do that is to avoid as many activities as possible that involve details."

"You mean like leading a Scout troop?" I asked quickly. (I knew how hard that had been for Dick the last year or so—and for me as well.)

"Yes, that's a good example of what I mean," was the answer.

"What about my job?" Dick asked.

"I'd say just play that by ear," the doctor replied. "If you have any problems, talk them over with your employer. If it becomes too troublesome, you might want to consider an early retirement." After a short pause he said, "Guess that's about all I have to tell you, Dick. You're free to go as soon as you get all your things together."

He nodded toward the nurse waiting nearby, and she took Dick into his room. He motioned for me to stay.

"Mrs. Atkins, I'm sure you understood by now that there is much more to this than I explained to your husband. We think this is all he needs to know right now. You will have to be the judge as to whether, sometime in the future, you feel that you should tell him anything more."

"But, doctor, there is so much that I don't understand about this. Until I came here, I had never even heard of it. What is going to happen to Dick? What should I do for him?"

Very patiently, he went into a fairly detailed explanation of what to expect. He cautioned me, several times, to try and save Dick from all the pressure and stress possible. He told me that I must be prepared to see him "losing ground from here on out."

Two particular statements still stand out clearly in my mind. Perhaps that's because they both aroused such strong feelings within me. The first was when he said, "There is a great possibility that your husband will become violent. If so, it will most likely be at you, for it is usually directed at the one closest to the patient." Inwardly, I rejected that idea completely. Not *my* Dick! I thought. He's too gentle, and he loves me too much.

The second statement: "We can't tell how long he will live. But if he lives long enough, he will probably have to be institutionalized." This time I found it extremely difficult not to say what I felt. Never! Over my dead body! I vowed inwardly.

We shook hands. He expressed his regrets: "Mrs. Atkins, I wish it could have turned out differently." Before he turned away, he told me that we were asked to stop by the Neurology desk before we left.

By then, the nurse had Dick's things all packed. She took us down on the elevator and to the proper desk, then said goodbye.

The Chief of Neurology, who had directed all Dick's tests, was a very busy man. But almost as soon as we arrived, he appeared. In his usual kind, compassionate manner, he wished us well. He said something in an aside to Dick that brought the first smile I'd seen on his face all morning. To me he said, "Remember, Mrs. Atkins, if there is ever anything I can do, I'm as close as your telephone."

After stopping at the business office, Dick and I went to pick up my things and to see the good people with whom I'd stayed. At last we were headed out of Gainesville and toward Fort Myers. I think we were both glad to be heading home.

We stopped before long for lunch. Dick only picked at his food, saying he wasn't hungry. When we were in the car again, he leaned his head back and closed his eyes. I noticed how pale he looked. "Honey, are you all right?" I asked.

"Oh, I still have a nagging headache," he admitted. I gave him a small pillow for the back of his neck, hoping that would help some. He kept his eyes closed but continued to move restlessly.

As much as I wanted to get home, it was easy to see that Dick was in no condition to make the trip in one day. I started looking for a quiet place where he could rest.

When I finally stopped the car, he sat up and asked, "Where are we? Why are we stopping?"

I explained that we were in Zephyrhills, a small town just off the highway. "Honey, there's no reason for us to hurry home. I think it might be a good idea if we stop here and get a motel room for the night—that way you could rest. Would you like that?"

"Oh, yes," he sighed.

He lay quietly on his bed for several hours, again with a wet cloth over his eyes. When I brought his evening meal, he sat up and ate—a little better than before. Soon afterwards, he got ready for bed, gave me a hug and said goodnight. It wasn't yet dark.

After all the noise and activity at the hospital, the room seemed strangely silent. In fact, I heard few sounds anywhere. In all those past days, there had been little free time. Now, there was too much—hours and hours before we could finally leave the next morning.

How those long hours passed is still not very clear. I cried some I know—and paced the floor. Several times I left the room to walk just outside. But mostly, I just *hurt*. And the more I hurt, the more mixed-up I felt. "I can't stand it, God! I don't know what to do! I love him! I need him! Oh, *please,* help us!" So went my silent screams.

Even as I cried out for Him to help, the whole thing seemed so hopeless and so final, I didn't see at all how He could. Yet, to entertain such negative thoughts tore at me, too, causing a deep fear that my faith was slipping away.

My love for God had been growing since my first encounter with Him, as a very young child. I had always trusted Him, and He had helped me through some difficult times—particularly the deaths of my parents, of my three brothers, two sisters-in-law, and a beautiful little niece, whom I had adored.

But this was different! This was Dick! And I loved him above all else in the world. Now he was ill—seriously so—though at times it was hard to believe. I knew all too little about his affliction, but what I did know seemed scary and unreal. The faith and trust that had upheld me throughout most of my life was beginning to seem unreal as well.

I slept little that night, but on our way home the next morning, I hugged one small bit of comfort to my heart. For, during the long and lonely hours in that motel room, I had begun to glimpse one very important truth: If I were to have the strength to meet what lay ahead, it would not be due in any measure to *my* efforts, but to God's mercy. I had come face to face with my utter helplessness, and knew that for me, *there was no choice but to depend upon Him.*

Such dependence, I hoped, would bring back the trust which I so sorely needed; and, like a warm blanket on a cold night, the assurance that He loved us and always would.

We were both glad to get home. Dick was acting more like himself all the time. In fact, when we pulled into our driveway and stopped, he rolled down the window, stuck his head out and called joyfully, "Hi! little house! We're home!"

Seven

The Truth and an Early Retirement

In Pain or Song

Shadow and sorrow I bring to Thee
Let not the clouds hide Thy face from me
    Though this my way is long
    And hidden love's sweet song
I'd follow Thee.

Peace, when it comes, is Thy gift to me
Gladness and joy then I offer Thee
    When heart is filled with praise
    This my soul's gift I'll raise
In love to Thee.

Sadness and joy both alike to Thee
If our intent is Thine own to be
    Let me, O Lord, be strong
    And give in *pain or song*
My *all* to Thee.

After a long weekend of rest, Dick returned to his job on Monday morning. In the following weeks I was glad, many times, not to be working. My doctor had recommended an extended leave of absence some months before.

I had been hospitalized twice that year. Both times Dick had stayed with his mother, who lived in a duplex apartment adjoining that of his sister and her husband in Fort Myers. Dick's father had died the week before we left for Shands.

Now with Dick working—or trying to—I had my hands full with managing a home and running interference for him. I had also become guardian for my invalid sister, who was now totally helpless, and I had moved her to a nursing home in Fort Myers.

As the months passed, Dick's departure time for work grew later and later. It took him longer to dress, and he often seemed confused about each thing he tried to do. In spite of my attempts to help him, he would forget his clip-board, or his pen, or an ad he had meant to work on. Then he would end up coming back home to look for them. By the time he got to the office, it was sometimes quite late.

Soon he was forgetting which clients to see on a particular day, or if he did call on them, whether or not they wanted an ad in the paper that week. I started making a daily list for him, suggesting that he check off the name of each person he called on, putting a "yes" or "no" beside it to indicate whether there was to be an ad or not.

"That's a great idea," he said. "I'll do it!" Some days it worked, but more often than not he forget to refer to the list.

When he could no longer remember what day it was, he asked me to get him a large desk calendar, so that he could mark off each day as it came. He insisted on doing it himself. But that didn't work either. He seldom remembered to check it.

Dick had always been on the friendliest of terms with his clients, and they enjoyed his calling on them. It was not long, however, until, bewildered by his actions, they began to realize that something was wrong. For example, one day he called on a used car dealer, sketched off the ad to the client's satisfaction, sat chatting for a few minutes, and then rose and said, cheerily, "See you next week!" With that, he wadded up the ad and threw it into the waste basket on his way out the door.

Not wanting to hurt him, a number of his clients told him that they could not longer find the time to see to the ads personally, and were forced to go to an ad agency. They urged him, however, to drop by and say "hello" whenever he was in the neighborhood. (I would not have known any of this except for a conversation with Dick's publisher—the same one to whom I'd talked before—who was genuinely concerned about what was happening to him.)

It soon became apparent that Dick was becoming more frustrated and unhappy in his work. He, of course, did not understand the real reason, but thought that if only he could find another job, things would be all right. So, he began searching for "something better." It broke my heart to see him poring over the help-wanted ads, and there was no way that I could refuse to type a letter for him each time he found something of interest.

Though he was no longer contributing much to his job, his employers didn't want to fire him. They hoped that I could talk him into a voluntary early retirement. But how? Deep down, I knew that was the only answer. But how could I tell him that? For years he had said, "I'm not going to retire when I'm sixty-five. I feel good and I like to work. I'm going to work until I'm seventy-five!"

In earlier days I had always replied lightly, "No matter when you retire, you'll never be bored—you have too many hobbies." But now? He continued to feel well, physically, and he was still in his mid-fifties. Even though I knew he should retire, how could I tell him, let alone convince him?

One of the jobs that Dick had applied for was that of manager at an Eckerd's Pharmacy which was being built in a new shopping center near us. Even though I realized what a good impression he usually made, I was not at all prepared when he came home one day, and announced with shining face: "Honey, guess what? Today they told me at Eckerd's that I might get the job of manager! Proud of me?"

"Oh, of course I am. I'm always proud of you." I paused, trying to think of what to say next. "But Sweetheart, do you think that's wise? Remember that the doctor said you should avoid as much detail as possible. There could be a mountain of detail in setting up a store like that."

He sensed my dismay and the light went out of his eyes. He then replied, a bit sadly, "Marguerite, I don't believe you have any confidence in me at all. You don't think I can do anything any more."

It was unbearable to hear him say that. I knew at once that the time had come—as the doctor had implied it might—when I had to tell him more. Intuitively, I felt that it was better for him to know the truth than to feel that I didn't care—or that I was against him.

"Oh, Dick," I managed to say over the lump in my throat, "maybe it would have been better if the doctor had told you what's really wrong."

"Then why don't *you* tell me? I've felt for a long time that you were holding something back."

"All right, Darling. Let's sit down and I'll tell you." My heart was like lead, for I had yearned so to spare him this pain. I do not recall the exact words of my explanation—only that I tried to make them gentle as well as truthful.

In the telling, I felt his varying emotions, as the changing expressions moved across his face. Once, I thought I detected a faint hint of relief. (And why not? At least he understood now that there was a reason for all that had been happening—that it wasn't his fault.)

When I finished, his eyes misted a bit, then he said, "Well, if that's the way it is, I'll stop looking for another job. I'll just keep this one and do it the best I can, as long as I can."

In the face of such an outwardly calm and brave acceptance of what must have been, to him, a shattering revelation, I lost my composure completely and rushed from the room. Though I had shed many tears since this terrible nightmare began, never in all that time had he seen me cry. I didn't want him to see me now, but he followed me at once into our bedroom, where I stood sobbing uncontrollably.

At first, when he took me into his arms, I tried to draw away. I had wanted so much to help him, and knew how much my words had hurt. He is the one who is ill. I should be strong for him—and just look at me! I thought. But his arms felt so good around me that I stopped struggling and clung to him until my sobs subsided.

He held me close, murmuring words of endearment. His manner was so loving that it took me a while to understand that he was trying to do more than soothe me. He wanted to strengthen me, as well.

From his own inner confusion, he was able to reach out to me, that day, with words of clarity and concern. "Honey," he said, "we must be brave. We have to meet all these little trials and tribulations courageously, and just keep on going."

Little trials and tribulations, indeed! I was overwhelmed by the strength and caring of this man who was my husband—this man, who at the very time he learned that his life was falling apart, found it in his heart to comfort me. By his selflessness I was both comforted and strengthened. The knowledge that he would not be able to remember, for very long, the sad events of that day, helped to ease my heart somewhat.

But above all else, I felt a sense of deep thankfulness, for the moment. For in that one brief and precious moment, God had transformed us both.

On our vacation to the Florida Keys that summer of 1972, part of my mind was occupied with how I could broach the subject of Dick's retiring. His employers were patiently waiting for me to talk him into it.

When I finally mentioned it, a few weeks later, Dick was not at all in favor of the idea. As I started to talk about it again, he—the eternal optimist—said, "Oh, Honey! Don't worry. It's going to be all right."

But before too long, it became apparent, even to him, that his best efforts resulted not only in confusion and frustration for himself, but extra work for those who had continually to correct his mistakes. It was painful to see his self-confidence dwindle. But only when that happened did he become willing to consider what he had resisted so strongly—an early retirement.

The fact that I had decided to change my leave of absence to the status of permanent (early) retirement may have helped a bit in his decision.

But for Dick, deciding to do it and getting up the nerve actually to go into the office and say it, proved to be two different things. The first time he planned to tell his employers, he came home admitting that he "just couldn't do it!" The second time, he came home early and said, "You know, it would be easier if you were with me. Let's drive back over to Lehigh, and I'll tell them today." By the time we got there, the office was closed. I knew that he felt both sorry and glad.

I kept on praying. Then one day, not long afterward, he burst into the house with his face beaming and cried, "Sweetie, I did it! I told them!"

"What did they say, Honey?" When is your last day?"

"They said I could take this whole week off. We're going to settle everything right after they get back from their Christmas vacation," he said jubilantly.

We had a lot to do in preparation for Christmas. We were expecting his sister and her grandson from Ohio, and of course his mother was to be with us, too. I found it a mixed blessing to have Dick home that week. He wanted so much to help. But, unlike other years, he found it difficult to remember what he was supposed to do. Or, if he did remember, seemed unable to do anything with the ease which used to be his.

One evening I watched him trying to wrap a medium-sized package, which needed to go to the Post Office the next morning. He had always been an expert at wrapping packages, but this time he seemed perplexed and very frustrated. I offered to help him and he flatly refused, saying, "I've been wrapping packages all my life, and I don't need any help!"

When he finished, I could tell that it would never reach its destination like that. Had I been wiser, I would have waited and re-wrapped it without his knowing, But, as had always been our custom, and without thinking, I pointed it out to him. This brought on a sudden and very unexpected outburst of anger: "Here! Then you do it!" he yelled. Before I knew what was happening, he threw the box with great force, just missing my shoulder. Tempers flared. For a moment we scuffled. Then, he rushed down the hall and slammed the guest room door behind him, leaving me in a state of utter turmoil.

Was this the beginning of violence which the doctor at Shands had predicted, and which I had not believed could ever happen? I was sickened, not only at what had happened, but at my response. *He* is ill, but what's my excuse? I asked myself. How could I possibly act like that? It would take me some years to accept the fact that no matter how much I loved God, or Dick, my reactions—especially sudden ones—would all too often be very human.

By the next morning Dick seemed to have forgotten the incident entirely, and I was thankful. Our Christmas, except for the haunting sadness in my heart, was a good one. I was touched when I saw what he had written to accompany a gift to me, which we had picked out together. It was a copy of *The New English Bible,* covered in dark blue leather. Inside, on a beautiful card showing the Madonna and Child, he had written (obviously with great effort, judging from the number of mistakes and smudges) these poignant words: "DARLING __ __ __ may this Bible Always be with You __ __ __ Use it forever to guide you LOVE DICK"

After Christmas, it was decided that Dick's last day on the job would be January 26. Much to everyone's surprise, he came down with a severe case of flu the previous week. Since he had never had it before, I wondered if the stress he was under had lowered his resistance. In keeping with their usual kindness, his employers paid him not only for that week, but a very generous severance pay as well.

To top it all off, he was given a farewell luncheon by the staff at the newspaper. His picture appeared in the next edition, along with a fine write-up that concluded: "At the luncheon held in his honor, Mr. Atkins was presented with rock-cutting equipment so that in his newly found leisure time, he can pursue a hobby in which he has been interested for years."

Dick was very pleased to get the rock equipment and spent much time in the following weeks reading and studying rock magazines, and planning what he would make. Sadly, the planning was about as far as it got. Before long, I noticed that he spent less and less time talking about it. When he abandoned it altogether, I was certain that he found the intricacies of it just too much. I remembered how the doctor had said it would be "downhill all the way."

Never once had I been able to accept that as a fact, but had kept on praying that God would heal him. Many others were praying for him, too.

Our summer proved to be a pleasant one, with a visit from Karen and her young son, Michael. I had told her that this might be the last summer that she could really enjoy being with her father. She thought Michael was old enough, at age seven, to store up some good memories about his grandfather. Little Michelle, who was younger, stayed at home with her father. We spent several days at the beach while they were with us.

A very special treat, that fall, was our three weeks in a wooded spot near Hendersonville, N.C. We particularly enjoyed the display of the changing colors and the magic moment when each fragile leaf would finally fall was a constant wonder to us. Dick, always an ardent nature lover, reveled in that time spent outdoors.

On our way home, when we were well out of the city of Atlanta, Dick insisted on driving. Ever since a Veterans Administration doctor had confirmed my suspicions about the danger of his driving (his reflexes were too slow, he explained) I had been fairly successful in keeping him away from the steering wheel. "Dick, all these years I've been the navigator and you've been the pilot," I had told him. "It's only fair that I take *my* turn driving. That way, you can enjoy the scenery."

He had accepted that, so far. But for some unknown reason he would not be put off this time. There was no way I could stop him—I could not forcibly restrain him. He got very upset when I tried to show him the route on the map, and closed his ears, informing me that he knew how to read a map.

He was so angry that I had to let him go almost twenty-five miles back along the route we had just traveled, before I thought he was calm enough to say anything. When I told him, as gently as possible, that we were headed back toward Atlanta, he answered quietly, "We are?" Coming to a service station not long after, he pulled in and said, "I'm a little tired—why don't you drive for a while?"

After we returned home, I went to the Highway Patrol Office one day, leaving him to visit with his mother and sister. I knew that was the year for Dick's driver's license to be renewed by a test. After explaining the circumstances to the officer in charge, he said "No problem! Just bring him in on his birthday (October 28th) and we'll make sure he fails the test, that way, he'll have to give up his license and he won't be able to drive anymore."

There has to be a better way, I thought on my way home. "Oh, God, please show me," I prayed. The last thing in the world that he needed just then, was to feel that he had failed again. I longed to spare him that.

The next week I hit on what turned out to be exactly the right idea. Upon inquiring at the office that carried our car insurance, I learned that with one driver instead of two, we could save some money on our policy. True, it wasn't much—only thirteen dollars a year—but Dick had always been a great one to save, and somehow I counted on the fact that he would not ask "how much?" He didn't.

"Honey, how would you like to save money on our car insurance?" I asked one day.

"Sure, how?" he answered. I explained and then told him that it seemed like a good idea, since I was doing most of the driving anyway. He readily agreed, and we went together to the Highway

Patrol Office where he voluntarily turned in his driver's license.

When he received a letter from the Department of Safety and Motor Vehicles commending him for being such a good citizen of the State of Florida, he was more than pleased. I breathed a sigh of relief as I thanked God for having taken us over one more hurdle on this rocky road of Dick's inevitable early retirement.

Eight

Ghosts and Little Green Men

A Spirit of Joy

Open for me the gates
    of Thy compassion
Cover me with the dew of Thy love
Temper for me all sorrow
    and suffering
And fill the crevices of my heart
    with mercy.

Thy compassion, Thy love
    and Thy bountiful mercy
Will awaken in me a spirit
    of joy . . .
I will lift up my voice in song
    O Lord,
And be filled with Thy peace
    forever.

It was to be expected that Dick would be restless after he gave up his job. So I began to look around for something that would help to fill the void. A friend of his, who was manager of a small furniture store, helped by giving him a part-time job, two half days a week.

Though his duties consisted of little more than cleanup work, it gave him a feeling of being involved. He was also glad to be earning some money again and delighted when I suggested he save it to buy something he might really want in the future. He was crestfallen, a few months later, when the store closed and his job fell through.

It taxed my ingenuity to find enough things of interest to keep him busy. He continued to feel well and strong, and had an abundance of energy.

We attended church together, as always, and he started going to the weekly prayer group with me. We went to the beach some days, and now and then saw an interesting movie. For a while, he enjoyed being a part of a senior citizens' harmonica band. (He had always played the harmonica and the guitar.) We even joined in some of the activities at the tourist center. With so many people around, no one knew whether you were a tourist or not!

Of course he was still interested in his rocks and fossils, and continued his attempts at whittling. I could tell he was losing dexterity in his hands. It filled me with dismay to see how the simplest things were becoming increasingly hard for him

Dick had always been painstaking and capable in whatever he did. Now, just the opposite was true. A case in point was taking the trash out to the street. He invariably dropped or forgot things, going doggedly back and forth, trying to get it done right.

In this, as in other matters, I found myself in an untenable position. Either I had to say something, and risk upsetting him, or go behind his back and do a job over, never knowing whether he would see me or not. Though I knew that his outbursts were due to frustration, they were directed at me. Trying to cope with this, on top of my fatigue, only exhausted me more.

I realized that Dick needed companionship other than mine. So two of his scouting friends agreed to come by occasionally, and take him to a meeting of the Scout Commissioners. This lifted his spirits, for he had been involved for years. He always came home happier and more relaxed.

Much of the time, however, he was extremely restless—so much so that I began looking around to find him another part-time job. Someone suggested Goodwill Industries. That was perfect. Their main purpose was to help handicapped persons by providing them with useful employment. And, as much as it pained me to acknowledge it, I knew by then that my beloved Dick was indeed handicapped.

He was very pleased to be working again. Even though it was only two days a week, it gave him something to look forward to and made his life more meaningful. Besides that, it gave me a much-needed reprieve, sometimes for rest, but more often, for necessary chores which were more easily accomplished while he was away. I was thankful for both of us, but could only wonder how long he would be able to carry on.

It was evident that he was growing more confused each day. Somtimes he would come into the kitchen during dinner preparation and ask cheerfully, "Sweetie, what can I do to help?" I always picked out something easy, like putting ice in the tea glasses. "O.K. Coming up!" he would say with his still-mischievous smile. Often he wandered away when it was half done, or at times, before he even began. Since it was not of vital importance and he was not aware of it, I let it go.

There were three particular areas, however, in which his confusion was of real concern, and which sometimes brought friction between us. One was the matter of brushing his teeth. He never seemed to remember. When I reminded him, his response was always, "Just a minute!" When I had to remind him several times, he was more than apt to say, "You don't have to tell me. I've been brushing my teeth all my life!"

Then there was the matter of his getting dressed. I had to begin laying out everything he would need. Before he was finally dressed, one item—or two—or three— would be missing. He never knew what he had done with them, nor, of course, did I.

This assumed major proportions one early Sunday morning,

when he had misplaced one thing after the other. I was relieved when we were safely in the car and on our way to church. I soon discovered that he was more upset than I had realized, for we had scarcely turned onto a much traveled boulevard when he demanded that I stop the car and let him out. I said, "Oh, Dick, *please!*"

Just than he grabbed the wheel, shouting, "Let me out!" In the midst of heavy traffic I managed to turn off onto a grassy knoll. My intention was to try and calm him, but as soon as the car slowed, he jumped out and slammed the door. By the time I could turn around and get the car back on the road, he had disappeared.

I searched and searched for him, driving slowly back and fourth between that point and home several time, but without success. I was filled with fear. Fear that he would not be able to find his way home, or worse still, that he might be hit by a car.

He found his way. When he finally arrived, hot and tired, he seemed to have all but forgotten why he was walking. *I* couldn't forget, however, and thanked God for his safety. Oh, dear God, I thought, such heartache all because we both got so uptight over his dressing!

Getting him to brush his teeth, and trying to see that he was adequately dressed were two ever–present concerns. But another began to loom larger.

If I had ever wanted to close my eyes to what was happening—to wake up and find it just wasn't so—it was during the following weeks. Dick started to speak of strange and unusual happenings in our house. When he first told me that there were "little green men" flying in and out of the bedroom windows, I thought he was joking. He convinced me he was serious, when he said that he *knew* what had happened to my diamond ring that had been lost. He declared that he saw one of "them" put it into a brown paper bag and then fly "right out of the window with it."

The "ghosts walking in the hall" caused us even more trouble. When Dick couldn't get me to agree that I'd seen them, too, he became indignant. "You know you see them," he claimed. "You just won't admit it!" Thus did our confrontations become not only more frequent, but more serious.

By then I knew that I needed help in handling these situations. But where to turn? Father Haynes had just been elected Bishop and was in the midst of a move to St. Petersburg. A local doctor had told me, concerning Dick's retiring, that it was none of my business and to "stay out of it!" I had already tried a counseling service. But when, early in our first session, the counselor interrupted my telling him something about Dick by saying, "I don't know why you're telling me all this . . ." I left, and never went back.

As I prayed desperately for guidance, Dr. Greer came to mind. I remembered how he had said, "If you ever need me, I'm as near as your telephone." But would he remember Dick? It was then nearing the fall of 1974, two and a half years since he was a patient at Shands. I decided to give it a try.

It was easier than I thought. He remembered Dick's case quite well. His suggestions to our problems were concise and clear. About his brushing his teeth, he said, "Make up a funny little song about it that will bring a laugh—tease him into it." I did, and it worked.

In regard to his getting dressed, he said, "Mrs. Atkins, try using the light touch as much as possible. If he puts on the wrong color tie, for example, let it go—it's not that important. Of course if he gets into the car barefoot, or with his bedroom slippers on to go to church, you'll have to say something—but laugh *with* him. Each time that he misplaces something, just matter of factly give him something else in its place. But whatever you do, in whatever situation, keep it light. That will cause less stress for him and also for you."

About the "ghosts and little green men" he said. "Mrs. Atkins, don't ever contradict him on that. He *does* see them. His mind is disturbed enough now that he can see them in the pattern of a drape, in a palm frond brushing across the window, or in moving shadows in the house. When he speaks of it, tell him that you're sure he sees them, but you haven't seen them, yet."

He ended by telling me that this was a long-term illness, and advised me to seek out any support I could, for I was going to need it (Mental Health Support Groups exist in almost every city today—but not then). He urged me to feel free to call him anytime. His advice helped, and for a while at least, tensions were lessened.

In spite of all our problems, my love for Dick grew rather than diminished. I had only to close my eyes to see the happy, carefree person that he used to be. In fact, upon occasion, he was much like the loving, caring husband that he had always been. Loving him, I yearned to help him. And I prayed constantly, that God, in His mercy, would give me the wisdom and the strength to do so.

Nine

A
Calculated
Risk

All For Thee

Do the birds answer Thy call—
Is that their melody?
Is the trilling and the billing
    All for Thee?

Are the clouds that sail above
Floating so fast and free,
But a cover as they hover
    Over Thee?

Do the flowers on the ground
Lifting their faces, see
In their swaying (or their praying)
    Only Thee?

Is the rain that finds its way
Through foliage green of tree
So refreshing, but expressing
    Love for Thee?

All of Nature seems ordained—
Whate'er its way may be—
To be praising, as it's raising
    Voice to Thee.

God of Nature, hear my prayer,
O help Thou even me
To surrender, as I render
    All to Thee!

When Dick's job at Goodwill began, it was a boon for both of us. It brought a semblance of order to our lives. In those early weeks he looked forward to Tuesdays and Fridays, when he worked from ten o'clock to four. He was always ready early, and seemed eager to go.

As time passed, I began to detect certain changes in his disposition—changes so subtle that it was hard to tell whether they were real or not. All too soon, however, his inner conflict became not only more obvious but more frequent. This resulted in mood swings that were not at all like him.

For one thing, he seemed almost obsessed by a need to find out everything he could about my activities while he was away. He wanted to know where I had been, what I had done and whom I had seen—*especially* whom I had seen.

This was so totally out of character that I wondered what was going on in his mind, what was behind this sudden concentration on my activities. It seemed to have a tinge of suspicion, or even jealousy. But Dick? Oh, no—never! I thought.

There were times when he would go from a cheerful mood to one of irritability, for no known reason. He fluctuated between moments of being very talkative and periods of deep silence, which I could not understand. Sometimes his spirit was upbeat, and at other times it was sad. But, often still, it was the dear and loving man I had married, whose gentle, caring spirit came through. I was thankful for those times. They were the joyful ones and I did everything possible to foster them.

Several times I reminded him that I was holding the money he earned for the time when he found something he especially wanted. That day came when he found a 19-inch color T.V., which was in perfect condition and very reasonably priced.

His driver knew about it and had taken him to see it on the way home. I could tell how excited he was. Our T.V. was a black-and-white and quite old. "This is it, Honey! This is what I want to get for us!" he exclaimed.

"Are you sure, Dick?"

"Yes, I'm sure," he answered quickly, "if it's O.K. with you."

"Of course it's O.K. with me, Sweetheart," I assured him. "It's your money and you can use it any way you like. You earned it— I've only been keeping it for you."

It had been a long time since I'd seen him so enthusiastic about anything. He kept telling me what a good T.V. it was, and what a bargain. (He was right, I am still using it.) More than anything else, I think, he was proud that he had paid for it out of money he had earned!

I was glad for that one thing, at least, which gave him so much pleasure and a sense of worth. For there were many things that brought him nothing but frustration. Of those, perhaps the one thing that bothered him most was his increasing inability to keep track of his things. Whatever he needed the most seemed always the hardest thing for him to find. But he was not one to give up easily.

Thus there was a constant conflict between his resolute will and the encroachment of the insidious disease. Because I was so close to the situation, I found myself, more often than not, caught up in this as in almost everything else that happened.

The sound of dresser drawers opening and closing had become almost as routine around our house as the humming of the refrigerator. It became so constant that it began to arouse within me feelings of dread. Each time, I knew it meant that Dick was looking for something else that he could not find.

He always refused any offer to help. His attitude continued to be one of dogged determination and independence. In this, as in all other circumstances, he would invariably declare, "You don't need to help me. I'll find it (or do it) myself!"

While I could not help admiring his indomitable spirit, there were times when, like a mother with a small child, it would have been much easier for me to do something or find something for him myself. In fact, at times, I feared that the sound of just one more dresser drawer opening and closing might bring out the scream that I felt inside.

One day in particular comes to mind—a day when everything seemed out of kilter. I was very tired. I had a nagging headache, my back hurt, and my nerves felt like tingling points of pain. In spite of my deep love for Dick, trying to cope was taking its toll.

When he finally decided, that afternoon, to take a nap in his hammock, which hung between two shade trees in our back yard, it seemed a good time for me to lie down and take a rest, too. I stretched out where I could keep an eye on him. In the quiet, I must have fallen asleep.

When I groggily came to, it was to a noise which at first I could not identify. Then, fully awake, I knew that it was Dick opening and closing dresser drawers again—at a faster rate and with greater force than usual. I might have recognized that as a sign of a particular frustration on his part, except for the renewed throbbing in my head and the nerves in my back which had set up their own little sadistic dance.

"Dick! Will you please stop that racket!" I cried as I rushed toward the bedroom.

He looked so startled. His face showed surprise, bewilderment, guilt and pain, all in one fleeting moment. He turned away from me and closed the drawer very softly, his shoulders sagging.

At the realization of how I had hurt him, I was conscience stricken. The pain in my heart, at that moment, exceeded all the others. I started toward him. He just stood where he was and looked at me sadly.

"Oh, Darling, you know I didn't mean to yell at you like that. I never meant to hurt you." I put my arms around him and looked up into his face, "Oh, please forgive me."

He stood stiffly erect for a moment. Then slowly—very slowly—I saw the softness return to his eyes. He put his arms around me and held me close, saying gently, "It's all right. Don't worry about it. You love God, and that's the most important thing. All the other things will take care of themselves."

I realized that once more, his inner spirit had somehow taken precedence over his ailing body and his disturbed mind. I was deeply moved by his generosity.

Though I had tried to accept my own humanness, I was grieved each time that I added outer conflict to that which he must wage within. This time was no different. So, as we stood holding each other, I prayed a silent but fervent prayer. I prayed that our Lord, in His infinite and loving compassion, would always give us comfort in the midst of conflict, and His peace, in spite of the pain.

When I realized that Dick no longer looked forward to going to work—that he seemed to dread rather than enjoy it—I called his supervisor. He confirmed what I had suspected. The simplest job they had now was too hard for him. Dick hadn't said anything because he didn't want to be labeled a failure—especially by me.

When I told him one evening, in a rather oblique manner, that he was retired now, and this job was something for him to do only as long as he chose, his countenance brightened at once. When I told him how nice it would be to have him home all the time, he said, "You really mean that?"

With a little reassurance he was convinced and so went back only one more day, in order to tell them that he was through.

I must admit to having a few qualms, for this meant that we would be together twenty-four hours a day. I wondered how I would be able to keep him interested and occupied all day, every day, for he was still quite active.

The hours of the day did prove quite long, sometimes. As time went on, it seemed that our lives began to center around three things: fishing, fossils and *fear*. Dick had a lifelong interest in the first two, and I wanted to encourage him all I could. The fear was mine. I couldn't seem to shake it and it began to color my days.

Dick was content to fish from the shore, and since there was a canal opposite us on one side, and the Orange River on the other, this presented no problem. But his continuing desire to look for fossils was another thing altogether.

His favorite "hunting ground" had always been an island out in the middle of the Caloosahatchee (the river of the long-ago Caloosa Indians.) He had, in the past, found some of his rarest and most treasured ones on "Beautiful Island" as it was called. He had his heart set on going back there again.

I knew that he would have to go up the Orange River and into and across most of the wide Caloosahatchee to reach "his" island, and I was fearful that he was no longer able to negotiate it.

While he thought only of the fossils he hoped to find, I was filled with an almost consuming fear when I thought of his taking his boat out alone. He was adamant about making it on his own as he had always done. I kept telling myself that because he preferred rowing his boat to using his motor, it should be safer. He had always been an excellent swimmer—a lifeguard in North Africa in World War II. But I was afraid he might become completely disoriented and get lost. The boat might tip over and he would swim in the wrong direction, or it would hit him on the head, knocking him unconscious, or . . . or . . . or . . .!

Each time Dick mentioned the island, I found myself making one substitute suggestion after the other. It was not long until he sensed my reluctance, and said one evening "You don't want me to go, do you? Well, I'm going tomorrow and you can't stop me!" Then in a gentler tone, "Aw, Honey, there's nothing to be afraid of. I can take care of myself." What could I say?

After he was sound asleep that night, I sat in the Florida room, looking at the stars in a very clear sky. The night was serene. But within me was a cauldron of fear and indecision. There was no person I could call on for counsel, so little was known about Alzheimer's then. I longed to make the right decisions as I tried to care for him, but often, very often, I wasn't even sure what the right decisions were. And when he made up his mind, as he had done about going to the island, there was little I could do about it, anyway.

"Oh, God, please help us—please keep him safe," my heart cried out that lonely evening.

I wasn't sure at first why, after crying out to God like that, my thoughts should suddenly turn back to a time, years before, when I hadn't even known Dick. I found myself thinking of my mother and of an almost-forgotten conversation I'd once had with her doctor.

My mother had always loved to fish and usually brought home a bigger catch than my father or any one of my three brothers. When, due to acute angina, her doctor suggested that the use of the rod and reel was too strenuous for her, she was undaunted. She would have my father drive her to a nearby lake or stream and position her lawn chair just at the water's edge, where she would fish with a cane pole.

I was very concerned for her, and one day, I approached her doctor, who was also a friend. "George, won't you please tell her not to do that?" I begged. "One of these days she's going to have a heart attack and fall in the water and drown!"

George looked at me kindly and said, "Marguerite, you know as well as I do how much your mother enjoys fishing. I can't tell her not to do it—that's the only real pleasure she has left." He looked straight at me, as he continued. "You know, there come times in life when we have to take a calculated risk, and I believe this is one of them." He paused and then said, "If she falls in the lake and drowns, at least she'll die happy!"

I had my answer—"a calculated risk." I knew then that I'd never again try to stop Dick from going out in his boat. And I had the sudden assurance that the risk wouldn't be all that great, anyway.

For, in surrendering Dick to God, I knew that He would surely go with him.

The next morning Dick began to assemble the things he would need for the day. As always, he did not want me to pack a lunch for him, but asked for "just a couple or three oranges and apples, and a thermos of water." That was all he had ever wanted on jaunts like this.

Because I knew he preferred it that way, I made no effort to help him carry his things down to his boat. My heart ached at the number of times I saw him plodding back and forth from our house, repeatedly crossing the street and a very large lot, to where his boat was tied up. I knew he was having a harder time remembering the things he would need, but he patiently made trip after trip.

Only when I saw him getting ready to leave without the bucket he usually took along for the fossils he hoped to find did I go flying after him. "Dick, Honey, wait!" I called.

He was happy that I had brought it and, giving me a quick hug, said, "You're my Sweetie. I'm going to bring you some good ones today. You'll see!"

When I saw the joyful glow on his face that day, I knew that in spite of the risk—the calculated risk—I would never try to hold him back again. I knew that just as surely as God watched over the birds and all that was a part of His creation, He would watch over Dick as well. My part was to let him go, pray for him during the hours he was away, and greet him warmly when he returned.

I had no way of knowing then that his trips to the island would be so few in number. I knew only that on that morning he seemed happier and more carefree than for a very long time—which was enough for me. I stood and watched him go. We waved to each other until he was almost out of sight.

Ten

The Matter
of Healing

That I May Trust

Open mine eyes
To see
What Thou wouldst have me see;
Open Thou my mind
That I may understand
What Thou dost will that I understand.

But when I cannot see
And if I should fail to understand
Grant me, O most merciful Lord,
An heart with which to love Thee
And to trust . . .
Always.

Dick made two more day trips to "Beautiful Island" within the next week. I prayed each time: "Into Thy hands I commend him," but found it much easier to say than to do. His excitement and joy were evident at first, but then, as with so many other things, he forgot all about it.

Much of the time now, he was restless and irritable—even to the point of sudden outbursts of anger. It would have been hard for him, I suspect, to have come up with a specific reason. I knew it was the disease. Each day became little more than a long string of hours to get through—hopefully without the explosion that I sensed was waiting to happen.

One blessing for me, at that time, was that Dick still slept so well. (I have learned that this is not always true of Alzheimer's patients.) I worried when he began to sleep so very late, not knowing whether to get him up or to let him sleep. Then I remembered that the doctor from Shands had mentioned that possibility when we talked on the telephone. His advice was now helpful.

"Let him sleep later," he said, "his body needs the extra rest. But get him up at least by nine, or ten at the latest. His brain also needs to be stimulated." I did what he said, for I was afraid that otherwise, his brain might atrophy at a faster rate.

But, because he did sleep so soundly, I found that I could get up and take an early morning walk beside the Orange River before he awakened. I loved being out when the breeze was cool, and the rays of the sun were casting their first faint hint of color on the rippling waves. Hearing the early songs of the birds, as they called back and forth to each other, lifted my spirits.

I often thought of an almost-forgotten line of a hymn: "This is my Father's world." I was strengthened in knowing that we, too, were a part of His world, and that He loved us. I clung to the hope that no matter what happened—no matter how bad things might become—God would continue to love us and be with us.

Aside from the outer struggle of trying to keep our daily lives somewhat on an even keel, another battle was going on within me. It had to do with the matter of healing. I had always believed in God's power to heal, and so had Dick. Some literature which had come into my hands recently, however, seemed to point toward an affirmative attitude as the chief pathway for the release of God's power in healing. Negative thoughts were not to be condoned, so went this line of reasoning.

Though I had always believed in God's love as well as His power, I had felt that He knew and understood things I didn't, and I was willing to leave it to Him. But now, I was assaulted by these new ideas, which resulted only in uncertainty and anguish. Was it because my thoughts were not affirmative enough? Was it because I could not say, and mean it, "I *know* he will be healed?" Was it because of a lack of faith on my part? Was it because of me that Dick had to suffer and die?

"Dear God," I cried, time after time, "is it *my* fault?"

Day by day coping was hard enough, but this new burden of uncertainty and guilt seemed more than I could bear. And there was no one with whom I could share it. Or so I thought.

In God's perfect timing, an announcement came, through the church, that there was to be a healing mission, Wednesday through Friday, November 13-15, 1974, at St. Mark's Episcopal Church in Venice, not too many miles north of us. It would be led by Emily Gardiner Neal, a leading figure in the Christian healing ministry, and a writer of several books on the subject. I had first learned of her some years before, when Father Haynes had handed me one of her books entitled, *The Lord is Our Healer*, and said, "Here, I think you would like to read this."

I read and liked the book and subsequently purchased and read another, *The Healing Power of Christ*, which I liked even more. But so much had happened since then, and I had been so bombarded in the meantime by the "affirmative–negative feeling" ideas, that what I had read in her books was pushed far back in my mind and all but forgotten.

It was not hard to talk Dick into our attending the healing mission. It was a break in the everyday monotony, for one thing. We would spend three days and nights in a motel in order to attend all the sessions and services. But more than that, I found that Dick had never quite lost the deep interest in spiritual healing, which had long been a part of him.

His interest in the subject had preceded mine. When we were in California it grew, and he often talked with our priest about it.

I will never forget how he came home from work, one day, and told me of a young secretary whom he had found in tears. She opened up to him, telling him about her four year old daughter. Exhaustive tests had been performed, and the child had been declared hopelessly retarded.

After assuring her that he and our priest would pray for her daughter, he asked her to pray with them, and set a time. At the appointed hour, Father Ken and Dick met in the church where they joined in specific prayers for the little girl.

I had all but forgotten about it when, a week latter, Dick burst into the house, an exhuberant look on his face. "Honey! Guess what? I called at the same office where the secretary was in tears last week, and—" He had captured my attention completely with his excitement and his look of utter joy.

"She was looking for me," he continued, "and was happy when I walked in. She said she had been hoping I would come!" It seemed that he couldn't get the words out fast enough.

"Honey, she took her little girl back and insisted on more tests and, you know what?" Here he paused for breath. "The doctors are very puzzled. They found that little girl perfectly normal!"

He hugged me in his excitement and joy. That was a long time ago, but I have never forgotten the happiness that shone on his face that day.

Although the mission in Venice was only ten years ago, strangely, I remember very little of what was specifically said in the more public sessions held there. I do remember that in the question and answer period I was relentless in my questions, and Mrs. Neal was equally direct in her answers, which were based for the most part on Holy Scripture. She had been dealing for years with those who had grave problems that tore at their lives, and her concern came through as completely uncamouflaged and real.

During the early part of the mission, the weight and the worry which had been gnawing at me, began to dissipate. Dick and I were happy as we lived two lives—one in the church, and another outside. The beach was nearby and we drove over several times to walk up and down—just out of reach of the frisky little waves.

Dick even found some fine sharks' teeth—Venice is noted for those. He had been there a number of times in the past for that very purpose, usually with a bevy of Boy Scouts. Though he did not completely lose his restlessness, he did seem in a calmer and more peaceful frame of mind.

I had asked for a conference with Mrs. Neal and was to see her immediately after the daytime session on Thursday. Two friends from home, who were also attending the mission, "kept" Dick while I went in to talk with her.

At first I felt very tense, but she soon made me feel at ease. I told her of Dick's illness and of our many and growing problems. She remembered him from the healing service the night before, when he was the first one to hurry to the altar rail, for the laying on of hands with prayer. She spoke of his eagerness and of the fine qualities evident in his face.

"He is God's child, without any doubt," she said. "I know from what you tell me that you both love God, and you may rest assured that you are loved in return." She paused and then went on. "Marguerite, we know that God's perfect will for Dick is *wholeness*. He taught us by His ministry on earth the importance of physical healing. But He also taught us that the healing of the body does not come first in importance, but wholeness, in the sense of holiness. This comes only through the complete adandonment of ourselves, or of those we love, into His hands."

There was a silence. Then she asked: "Can you relinquish Dick into the hands of Him who loves him more, even than you?"

After a slight hesitation, I said, "I want to, I have *willed* to do just that. But . . . my feelings often get in the way."

She nodded, as she said gently but firmly, "It's your *will* that matters most. God will take care of the feelings."

We talked for a few moments longer and then she prayed. For the first time in a very long while, I felt comforted and strengthened. I knew then, beyond any shadow of a doubt, that no matter what happened, "All things (would indeed) work together for good to those who love God." (Romans 8:28) And that meant Dick, and me, for we loved him.

I felt a deep certainty, not only that God loved us, but that I was not losing my faith and that there was no need to blame myself for what was happening to Dick. I resolved to pray more fervently than ever for understanding, for love, and always for a more perfect trust.

After the final service on the last evening, Dick raced ahead of me and I saw him shake Emily's hand as he said something to her. By the time I reached the outside door, others had claimed her attention.

When she saw me leaving, she broke away for a moment to speak to me. "I want you to remember, Marguerite, that you and Dick will be very much in my prayers." Then she took my hand and said earnestly, "If there is ever any way that I can help, please let me know. Keep in touch."

I thanked her, never dreaming how soon I would take her up on her offer.

Eleven

Devastating Decisions

Small Part

Most loving Lord
I know
This pain of mine
Is but a small part
Of Thine
But it is all
I have
To offer Thee.

If Thou
Canst not take
It from me
Then make
It a part
Of the pain
Of Thy heart
And use it for another
For some other
Child of Thine.

Use it today
For someone
Who is alone
And forlorn
I pray.

I had hoped that with the three days away, our life together would improve. It didn't. Dick had seemed more like himself while there, but driving home Saturday morning, he was uncommunicative and moody. When we arrived, well before noon, he got out of the car, slammed the door, and walked toward the house without a word. I was puzzled and wished, as I had countless other times, that I could know what was going on in his mind.

I wondered even more that afternoon, when I realized how he was silently watching me every minute. He seemed determined not to let me out of his sight. My attempts to talk with him, to draw him out, were futile.

After we were ready for bed that night, he took a pillow and stretched out on the living room floor. "Honey, it's time for bed," I told him. No answer. "Dick, aren't you coming to bed?"

He sat up and said, "No, I'm going to stay right here."

"Why?" I asked, completed baffled.

"This way I can tell if you get up after you think I'm asleep, and try to sneak out to meet that man you've been seeing. You don't fool me any. I know what's been going on!"

"Oh, Dick, you know that's not true." This was the most unexpected blow yet; he had always maintained that he trusted me more than anyone in the world. "Please, Dick, won't you come on to bed?" His answer was to turn his face away and close his eyes.

I waited for a moment, then turned off all except one small night light, and went into the bedroom. I had a virtually sleepless night. Several times I got up to check on Dick, covering him with a light blanket when it turned a bit cooler after midnight.

The next morning, being Sunday, we dressed in preparation for church. Dick was moody and silent. This mood continued until we were well on the way. Then, like a volcano erupting, his pent-up feelings and accusations began to pour forth. Trying to talk with him, or to deny any of the allegations, about which he seemed so positive, was of little use.

It was just as we drove into the church parking lot and I stopped the car, that he literally shouted "You're nothing but a no-good, low-down tramp!" Before I even realized it, my right hand left the wheel and hit his face with a stinging, back-handed slap. I was crying and he was furious. "Don't you ever do that again!" he yelled.

"And don't you ever call me that again," I cried. With that, I was out of the car and running toward the parish house, dissolved in tears. I found seclusion in the small parlor, which was seldom used at that hour.

Only one person came in—a friend of mine. Upon learning what had happened, she went out to stay with Dick until my tears were under control and I felt able to go and take him with me into the church.

In my heart was a turmoil of pain, whether because of Dick's words or my response, I wasn't sure. I understood that he was no longer responsible for his actions, and felt that I had handled the crisis badly. Feelings of regret filled my heart. I could only hope that, since our Lord had chosen to share our humanity, He must surely understand and forgive such a human reaction as mine.

Receiving Him in the Holy Eucharist that morning kept me from being completely overwhelmed. My prayers were unspoken ones, from deep within my heart.

Dick never mentioned the incident, that day or the next, nor did I. He looked so sad and lost that my heart ached for him. He tried to do nice little things for me, insofar as he was able. I tried, also, to make him feel better in every way possible. I wanted very much to lift his spirits.

I thought much about the peace that we had both felt during the mission, such a few, brief days before, and wondered why it was so elusive at home.

To my surprise, he slept on the floor again on Tuesday night. This time we did not discuss it at all, but I felt very uneasy. When I went into the living room a few hours later to cover him with a blanket, he had curled up on the sofa. He didn't awaken, and I lingered a few moments. It touched me deeply to see how, in sleep, his face took on the gentle, peaceful look of the Dick whom I had always loved.

He carried a touch of moodiness with him into the next day,

but by Thursday things seemed to be getting better. That evening
he seemed happier than for a long time. We both enjoyed our hours
together out in the Florida room, first watching T.V. and later
looking at the moon and the stars. Together we watched the clouds
as they drifted lazily over and around them.

Dick was very loving. It felt so peaceful to sit close to him and
I hated to leave the comfort of his arms. But it was growing late
and so we began to close up in preparation for bed.

We had meant to keep Little Red our cat, in the utility room
that night, but he escaped, and try as I would, he kept out of reach,
refusing to come in.

I gave up and went into the bathroom to brush my teeth. The
door was ajar. Dick was still trying to coax Little Red inside, when
I called out to him, "Never mind, he'll be all right. He'll come in
later on." Then I added with a laugh, "That crazy little cat doesn't
know a good home when he's got one."

Suddenly Dick appeared at the door. His eyes were blazing as
he said vehemently, "And I know someone else who doesn't
appreicate having a good home—you! You have a good home and
a good husband, but that's not enough for you. Oh, no! You have
to sneak around behind my back and go out with another man!"

I don't know what was most startling, his dreadful change of
mood, the look on his face, the tone of his voice, or the words he
hurled at me. I began to tremble as I started to speak. But before
I could say anything, he grabbed me and shouted, "I won't put up
with it any longer! Do you hear?"

With one part of my mind I knew that this was the violence
that had been waiting to happen, a possibility which I had never
wanted to consider, and yet had feared for so long. I didn't have
much time to think, however, for I found myself locked in a physical
struggle with Dick, and more frightened than I had ever been in my
life.

Dick was not a big man, but he was well built. His years of
swimming and camping, and his twice-weekly workouts at the "Y"
had made his muscles very strong. I was no match for him. Try as
I would, I could not shake the grip he had on my upper arms. He
maneuvered me into the bedroom and threw me on the bed, as he
said, "I'll show you! I'm going to beat you to a pulp!"

With a supreme effort, I managed to break away, scooped up
my purse and car keys from a table by the door, and ran for the car.

I knew I had to get out of there, but Dick was right behind me.
He grabbed my purse and shouted, "Oh, no you don't!" I still had

the car keys in my hand, and managed to get into the driver's seat. Dick planted himself in front of the open door.

"Get out of that car!"

"No, Dick."

"Then move over!"

"No!"

He stood, glaring at me, still in front of the car door. After a moment of silence, I said with more conviction than I felt, "You'd better move away, Dick. If you don't I may have to knock you down. I'm driving out of here." (I've often wondered what would have happened if he had kept on standing there—escaped from the other side, I suspect. I do not believe I could have hurt him.)

Fortunately, he moved back. I quickly closed and locked the car door, backing out so fast that I almost ran into a deep ditch. I drove away with him still standing there in his pajamas, my purse clutched tightly in his hand.

I left him alone. For the first time in years I left him *alone*. With me went the picture of his face—a face etched with vestiges of the anger he had felt, combined with puzzlement and pain, and just a touch of fear. I loved him, and yet that night, I had to leave him.

But without money, or even a driver's license, where would I go? "Oh, God," I sobbed as I drove away. "Oh, God, *please*, please help us!"

After driving aimlessly around for a while, I decided to go to Dick's mother's. It was with reluctance that I did so. But she will *have* to know tomorrow, I thought. The sleepless night that I spent, fully clothed, on the studio couch in her apartment, was scant preparation for what the next day would bring.

When Dick's sister and her husband saw our car in Mom's driveway so early the next morning, they came over to see what was wrong. They drove home with me, to see how Dick was, and hopefully, to retrieve my purse with driver's license, wallet, and checkbook. We all agreed that the time had come to seek outside help for him.

Dick was almost as keyed up as the night before. I found my wallet, tucked between the folds of a blanket in a bedroom closet.

But the purse could not be found. I feared that in his anger the night before he might have thrown it into the river or the canal.

Before we left, I made arrangements with a good friend across the street to watch Dick each time he went outdoors, and to call his mother every half hour or so. I would place frequent calls to Mom—my only way of keeping in touch.

Shortly after nine I started out by going to the Veterans' Administration office, only to learn that the Veterans' Service Officer was out of town for the day. I was unsure of where I should go next, but decided to go to the Social Welfare office and ask. They gave me directions to the Mental Health Clinic. That proved easy to find as it was housed in the former rectory of St. Luke's Church.

After I had explained our problem to the assigned social worker, she advised that I have my husband hospitalized that day. She said the kind of evaluation he needed could best be done in the psychiatric ward of the hospital.

She typed my "statement" and asked that I read it carefully before signing. She told me that it would then have to be signed by Dick's doctor, our lawyer, a judge, and finally by an official in the sheriff's office. They would pick him up, since we lived outside the city limits. Faced with all that was involved in having him "committed" made it a devastating decision. I almost decided to back out. But remembering the events of the evening before, I knew that this had to be done. I signed.

During that day I did a lot of waiting, since I had no appointments. It was no trouble getting the signatures of the doctor and the lawyer—they were aware of the situation already. But after waiting at the courthouse for the judge's secretary to type up the proper forms for him to sign, she said, "I think we can process this in about three weeks."

"But that won't do!" I cried in dismay. When I explained the urgency of the situation, she went to the judge's chambers and interrupted him long enough to explain matters, and to get him to sign the commitment papers.

Last of all, I went to the sheriff's department, where I had to wait almost two hours for two plain-clothes deputies to arrive. They were assigned to follow me home and to take Dick to the hospital emergency room, through which he would be admitted. It was then almost five o'clock.

When I pulled into the driveway at home, the deputies were right behind me. Dick met us at the carport door, glad, I think, to see someone after what must have been a lonely night and day. The deputies, at my request, told him only that they had come to take him to the hospital. He willingly got into their car.

By the time I reached the hospital and went through all the admission procedures for him, Dick had already been taken upstairs and assigned a bed. Upon arriving finally at his ward, he greeted me joyfully. He was in a cheerful, attractive room, in the almost brand-new psychiatric wing.

We sat together on his bed as he tried to tell me all about it. Then, with his arm around me, he asked wistfully, "Honey, have you been out with that man?"

As gently as possible I answered, "No, Sweetheart, I haven't, and I won't—ever. So you don't need to worry about that anymore."

"That's good," he said, reassured at least for the moment.

When I returned that evening he seemed glad to see me and proudly walked me up and down the hall, and to the therapy room and the day room. The nurse told me, as I left, that he had said I was his sister. That way he could enjoy being with me, while telling them of all the bad things his wife had done. She said this was not uncommon when someone was in such a disturbed state of mind.

It was the Friday before Thanksgiving when Dick was admitted to the hospital. Though he was mentally confused when he entered, he seemed in good shape otherwise. But that changed rapidly.

On Saturday, I could see that he was deteriorating physically. During the day he went from shuffling barefoot up and down the hall to being tied into a wheelchair with his head thrown back and muttering about things that had happened many years before. By Sunday evening I found that he had been moved to a room across from the nurses' station. They had a catheter on him and he was tied in bed, thrashing about and completely incoherent.

With concern so deep that even now it is painful to remember, I called Bishop Haynes in St. Petersburg. He had known and worked with a number of the psychiatrists during his ten years in Fort Myers. I told him of Dick's condition and the fact that the admitting doctor had not given me time enough to explain Dick's diagnostic history. He only wanted to know the immediate reason for his being there. I feared that the word "violence" might have resulted in Dick's having been overdosed with drugs, and I knew that he didn't tolerate medications well.

The Bishop advised me to change doctors and suggested the name of one he held in high esteem. He said we would talk on his visit to Fort Myers, two days later.

I called the social worker at the Mental Health Clinic early

Monday morning, and asked what I had to do to change doctors, telling her my preference. The quick reply was, "You've just done it, Mrs. Atkins. All you have to do is request it—we will do the rest."

A few days later, Dick's new doctor asked me to drop by his office. Among other things he said, "In all my forty years of practice, I have never seen a patient so allergic to drugs." Then he explained his plan for quick withdrawal, and how it was working. Gradually Dick was back, physically, to his normal self.

The first evening of Dick's hospitalization, I returned home to find the house a shambles—furniture moved, bookcases emptied, and waste baskets overturned (the result, no doubt, of his unsuccessful search for my purse). I went methodically through the next two weeks, numb with grief and uncertainty.

A lifelong friend, who was a nurse, came from a nearby city to be with me for a few days, and that helped. It was she who, upon insisting on doing the carpets for me one day, found my purse hidden under the vacuum cleaner in the utility closet.

She was also standing by when I was called to a meeting of Dick's doctor, his social worker and chief psychiatric nurse. There I was told that the psychiatric wing was for a two-week evaluation only; I must decide within a few days where I wanted him placed.

"You mean he can't come home?" I asked.

"Mrs. Atkins," the doctor answered, "that would not be safe for either of you right now. In his present state of mind he could kill you and never even know or remember that he had done it."

Then the social worker spoke up. "You have two choices, Mrs. Atkins: a nursing home, or G. Pierce Wood Memorial Hospital, in Arcadia. That is a state mental hospital," she continued, "but an excellent one."

"What about the future? Will he ever be able to come home?"

"That depends upon how he gets along," I was told.

The next day my friend and I drove to the hospital—about forty-five miles away. With what we learned of the place from the chaplain, along with the good things Bishop Haynes had told me about it the day we had talked, I leaned toward G. Pierce Wood. I liked the idea that it had a gymnasium and a swimming pool and hoped that Dick would be able to use them.

My friend had to leave the day before Thanksgiving and I missed her. The wife of another patient, who, as I did, visited her husband during both afternoon and evening hours, invited me home with her for a Thanksgiving meal in the late afternoon. It was good to be with someone who felt and understood the distress of a situation like ours.

When I finally told Dick's doctor that I would agree to his being placed at G. Pierce Wood (another devastating decision), I was told that he would be transported by van on Friday, December sixth— exactly two weeks from the day he had first been hospitalized.

I saw Dick on the evening before he was to leave. At that time I was informed that I should wait at least until Sunday to visit him in his new environment.

During those long days of waiting, the cries of my heart were continuous. I could only hope that God, in His compassion, would be able to unravel the strands of pain and longing, of loneliness and fear, for that was all I had to offer Him.

Twelve

God is in Charge

A Tiny Bird's View

On the steeple's stone cross sits a tiny bird
    Surveying the world afar:
He looks to the south and he looks to the north
    Toward a new half-moon and a star.
Though he seems oblivious to all that's around
    As he silently perches there,
The wakening life of the early eve
    Is to him most passing fair—
For he easily views from his throne on high
    What we groundlings can never see:
All the earth and the sky and the hill beyond
    To the topmost leaf of a tree.
He sits comfortably balanced, serene and at peace,
    Wondering why humans don't know
That *God* is in charge—that He loves the *whole world*—
    Including the people below!

"Wait! Don't leave me! I'm coming! Oh, Honey, *please! Wait for me!*" These were the cries that assaulted my ears and tore at my heart as I walked woodenly away from the building and toward the parking lot.

I had just left Dick after my first visit to him as a patient at G. Pierce Wood Hospital. He had not been allowed to leave the "receiving ward," and there were so many people milling around, and so much noise, that our visit had been most unsatisfactory.

The last sight I had of him was his struggling with a guard as he tried to follow me. My heart was filled with pain. The memory of the distress on his face as I left him caused an agonizing cry within me, "Oh, dear God! What have I done to him?"

The chaplain had explained that all incoming male patients would be received into that particular ward, with bars on the windows and guards at the doors.

"You will think on your first visit," he said, "that nothing is being done for him. But trained nurses, aides, and social workers— male and female—will be on duty, watching him every minute, and making copious notes. That is the way they can decide where, or in what building or program, each patient should be placed." Then he hastened to add, "Try not to let it get to you. Remember his stay in that building will be brief."

But it *had* gotten to me. On the way home, I hardly talked to the friend who was with me. The sobs were beating to escape, but I was able to hold them in until I reached home. My heart was numb with grief, the pain more lacerating than ever before. It was all but unbearable each time I remembered his cry: "Honey, wait! Don't leave me!"

The house seemed more empty than at any time since he had

left home, two weeks before, and another sleepless night kept me tossing. Worst of all, I found it impossible to pray.

The hours and days loomed before me like a great abyss. How would I fill the time? I knew I would continue to visit my sister at Shady Rest nursing home and keep on with my monthly service there as well as my church duties. But since I planned to visit Dick only on Sunday, Wednesday and Friday afternoons, that still left too many hours to fill. I was not prepared. What kind of life could I possibly have without my loving, laughing Dick?

Upon my next visit on Wednesday, I learned that he had first been placed in an "open ward" (without locks), but by the time I arrived had been moved again to a locked building. It was for his own safety, I was told. He had spent so much time "wandering" on the spacious grounds that they feared he would reach a nearby highway, and possibly be hurt.

When I saw Dick that day he was shuffling, head down. My heart sank. Though I took him out for a walk and to the canteen, there was no communication whatever. I felt sure that he must be on some medication, again, which he could not tolerate, and resolved to talk with his new doctor about it. I was heartsick.

I did talk with his doctor—several times during the following weeks—but it seemed to do little good. He was convinced, even after what I told him of Dick's earlier experience, that he was on the right track. I found it hard to trust Dick to this doctor, who seemed so determined to keep him on medication that I felt sure was making him worse.

During that early period, it was a numbing experience each time I visited him. He had always been so active and well, filled with a particular zest for living. To see him now brought a hurt that was almost too much to bear.

Finally, I went to his doctor once again to try and talk with him. His response was an exasperated question, "What is it you want me to do?"

"Take him off that medication he's on and let him be himself, as nearly as possible!" I cried.

"And what if he becomes violent and hurts someone? You could be sued, you know!"

"I don't believe that will happen," I said. "I'll take my chances." He made no promises.

I felt lost under the weight of worry, frustration and pain, and soon began to realize that *my* need for help—though of a different nature—was almost as great as Dick's. It was at some point in that period of distress that my thoughts turned to Emily Gardiner Neal. I remembered what she had said the fall before, at the end of the healing mission. "If there is ever any way that I can help, please let me know. Keep in touch."

Having no doubt that she had meant it, I wrote her a long letter. Then the sense of despair became so overwhelming that it seemed too long to wait. I called Calvary Episcopal Church in Pittsburgh, where she then worked, asking that she call me back, collect.

She called, sooner than I had expected. I felt as grateful as if I had been drowning and she had thrown me a rope. (It was to be only the first of many letters and calls which literally helped to hold my head above water in the difficult years to come.)

I cannot remember all of that conversation, but much of her counsel proved so helpful that it is still fresh in my mind.

She stressed, as she had done before, the importance of relinquishing Dick into God's hands, in this and in every situation. "You must continue to offer him—and yourself—up to God," she said. "Words are not necessary. It's what's in your heart that matters." Then she spoke about the problem with the doctor, "Remember that it is God who is really in charge. Keep on trying to get the doctor to understand about Dick's allergy to medication. Do what you feel led to do, but *trust* that God can charge his thinking and guide him aright."

We talked a few more minutes about other things that were troubling me. She assured me of her continued prayers and urged me to write anytime I felt the need for she would understand.

Then, just before hanging up, she said, "And, Marguerite, whenever you find it hard to pray, try a bit of thanksgiving for the good years you had with Dick."

Soon after that, I was waiting in Dick's building for the nurse to bring him out, when the doctor saw me and came right over. "Have you seen your husband since we last talked?" I told him I hadn't. (I had been away more than two weeks, due to illness.) His face was animated as he said, "You won't know him! I decided to cut his medication in half and there were no bad effects. Now he is off it entirely and you'll be happy at the change."

At that moment the door opened and the nurse came out, holding Dick by the hand. She was smiling.

I hurried toward him, searching his face as always. There, for the first time in months, I saw a flash of glad recognition. On his lips a slow smile began to form. An inexpressible joy filled my heart. As I embraced him, he hugged me back! His arms felt so good around me.

When we went outside that day, he did not shuffle, he walked—and his head was up. He was more alert, and seemed actually to listen to the birds, which he loved so much.

This did not change the course of the disease. I understood that. But it was good to have him back to the best that he could be. As we walked hand in hand, I prayed that God would always help me to remember that He was in charge—that I might truly learn to trust Him.

Then my heart whispered silently, "Thank You. Oh, thank You!"

———————

To visit Dick in a locked building, no matter how good the reason, was a hurtful thing. He had always been such a free spirit! Though I kept trying to relinquish him into God's hands, often I found myself, instead, struggling to call down His power for Dick's healing. I wanted to trust God, but it seemed so difficult to accept the fact that he might never live at home again.

Accepting was not as easy as I had always thought. In fact, even praying to accept was becoming all but impossible for me. This became very clear when I realized that an old and favorite prayer of mine—the Suscipe—used for many years was now omitted from my prayers. It had been for years a means of expressing to God my deep desire to belong fully to Him. But now, the words stuck in my throat each time I tried to pray them.

> "Accept, O Lord, my entire liberty, my memory, my understanding and my will. All that I am and have thou hast given to me; and I give all back to thee to be disposed of according to thy good pleasure. Give me only the comfort of thy presence and the joy of thy love; with these I shall be more than rich and shall desire nothing more."

It was not that my desire to belong wholly to God had lessened. On the contrary, it seemed to grow. But now, the implications of that prayer appalled me.

What if I should be confined, like Dick, never again to be able to go when or where I chose? Or if I should lose those precious memories of the richest part of my life? How could I be willing to lose all understanding, when it was so clear what such a loss meant, not only to him, but to me? And how could I continue to pray— and mean it—that God would take my will when it might mean that I could no longer decide anything for myself, but be subject, as Dick was, to the wishes and directions of others?

To verbalize that prayer by asking God to take those things from me, presented, for the first time, possibilities too dreadful to contemplate. I couldn't—I just couldn't—pray that prayer.

The bleakness within me was matched only by the somberness of the outward circumstances over which I had so little control.

True, I occasionally found myself able to look up as some of the clouds parted a bit. There were brief but sporadic flashes of Dick's old humor, and I learned that he was beginning to be loved by the patients and the staff. But the nurse informed me, also, that he had become incontinent, and it was apparent that his speech and vision were beginning to be affected.

His ability to remember seemed almost nonexistent. He did not recognize Karen when she came from Ohio to visit us in that early spring of 1975. And while I spent two or more full afternoons with him each week, he no longer knew my name. He seemed neither to anticipate my visits nor to remember them afterward. That hurt, of course, but I was glad for him since it meant that he would not suffer over our separation. He did seem to sense, somehow, that I was there especially for him.

Although we had known for seven years that Interstate 75 would take our home, it came as just one more blow when it happened less than four months after Dick was hospitalized.

Leaving that home with its years of wonderful memories was a wrenching experience. I found a new home in a lovely area about a half mile away. It was built by the same contractor and was quite similar to ours.

The medical staff had determined by then that Dick could begin coming home for his birthday, Christmas and overnight every month or so. Hopefully, having a home so similar and with the furniture placed much as it was before, he would not notice the difference. He didn't. It was I who found the move so difficult. For me it was a low, low time.

I prayed for God's strength to keep going, when it seemed

impossible to go on any longer. The loneliness in a now-silent house—whether old or new—seemed unendurable. The sharpness of the pain when I was with Dick, and the tears through which I sought to drive each endless mile home, made up my existence for a very long time.

The days were long, and the nights continued to be broken and restless. I wanted to believe, as Emily had said, that God was in charge. I found myself saying it over and over: "God *is* in charge. I *know* He is in charge." I yearned to believe—for how else could I endure?

From the depths of my distress, the cries of my heart were frequent; "God, please help us. God, help him! Oh, God, help me!"

Thirteen

His
Ministry(?)

Thoughts of My Beloved

Deep, deep within my heart
Thoughts of my beloved:
Loving him
And longing for his presence
As he *was*—

When eyes spoke
Of love and understanding
And the touch of his hand
Was both gentle caress
And strength to lean upon.
His was a life
Of loving and of giving
Not only to me
But to all who had need of him.
He loved the small creatures
Was humble
And worshipped God.

Now the outer man is changed
But, somehow I know
His spirit remains the same.
How else could his eyes light up
When he sees me
Though he cannot call my name?
And how could it be that he smiles,
Snaps his fingers to music,
Shows the same kindness to others
And is loved
By those who must live as he lives
And by those who give him care?

Deep, deep within my heart
Thoughts of my beloved:
Loving him still,
And longing for his presence
As he *is*!

It was at that particularly low time when, not knowing how much longer I could hold on, there came a ray of light. I learned that a healing mission was to be held soon in an Episcopal church in Tampa, led by Emily Gardiner Neal. It was over a year since the mission that Dick and I had attended together and about nine months since my first frantic call to her. We had "kept in touch."

By then I had learned more about healing missions, and how demanding they were on those who led them. I understood that there was no time for social visiting, but knew, also, that Emily was much in prayer at such times. She had conferences with individuals when or if she were led to do so.

My hope, of course, was to talk with her. But I felt that should this not happen, attending the mission would be helpful in itself, and so decided to go. I wrote her a note telling her of my plans to attend.

We met in passing during the early part of that first day of the mission. Emily said that we could talk for a short while after the morning session and to wait for her. I did, and we found a quiet spot in one of the Sunday School rooms.

After answering her query as to Dick's condition, I spoke of something that had been burning in my heart and mind for a long while. "Emily, I read of so many people who have been healed, physically, in answer to prayer. Then there are others who have received what some speak of as the ultimate spiritual healing—death and the nearer presence of God. But Dick has received neither. Where is he? In limbo?"

Her answer came quickly. "Marguerite, you don't think for one minute that God would desert someone who loved Him as much as Dick did, do you?" My assent was somewhat reluctant. She continued, "I'm going to tell you something and I want you always to remember it. *The spirit never ails and the spirit never sleeps.* You must understand that there are things going on now between Dick's spirit and the Spirit of God that he may not fully realize, and that you may never be able to see. But you've got to believe they're happening!" Those words would comfort me many times over.

When I mentioned how concerned I always became at being "down"—wondering if that were a sin, her reply was reassuring. "That happens because you love, and you are human. God does not expect you to be pure spirit—yet!" And about my being so super-sensitive: "Let God take that from you, He *can*."

Then, very hesitantly, I told her of the prayer that had become so impossible for me to pray. While it had loomed so very large to me, she cut to the heart of the matter at once. "If you cannot willingly offer Him those parts of yourself now, just ask Him to make you willing. He can, you know, not in the same way as for Dick, or anyone else, but in His way for *you*."

Then she offered further words of caution. I was glad to listen, not only because she understood my needs, but because she was a trained, experienced and prayerful counselor. "You must conserve your energy, Marguerite. This is for Dick's sake as well as for your own. As a way of lessening the pressure, try to seek diversion of some kind, especially with other people—with friends."

Urging me not to be over-scrupulous—which she knew by then was one of my hang-ups—she suggested that it might be well for me to keep my spiritual rule (Bible reading, prayer and meditation) simple. "It's sometimes better," she explained, "to add to a shortened rule when you have the strength, than to make it so demanding that you worry when it's impossible to keep."

"One last thing," she said, "pray always for God's peace." Her words were strengthening at a time when I needed to be strengthened. Just before we parted, she offered up a prayer, simple yet moving. It lifted my spirits and brought a surge of thankfulness to my heart.

Upon my return home I thought much about the things we had talked about, and especially began to cast about in my mind for things to do that would help to lessen the pressure. "Diversion" for me at that time would have to be something I enjoyed doing, and yet would not take too much time or energy.

I began to accept a few speaking engagements from various church groups, both in Fort Myers and in other towns. This had always proved stimulating and spiritually rewarding.

The richest experience that came my way, however,—the most

unexpected "diversion"—was my involvement with a Vietnamese family, who had only recently arrived in our town. The mother, her brothers and other older ones bagan to call me "Mom." The three girls called me BaNôi, which means grandmother in Vietnamese. During the two years they were here, we became very close.

Though Dick was never far from my thoughts, I cherished the time spent with such dear people. I shall always remember their gentle kindness, not only to me but to him on his visits home and when they went with me to see him in the hospital. There is still a bond, though they now live in a distant state.

As the months passed, God was patient. He eased the pain of what was happening by giving me time, not to get used to it—I could never do that—but to accept what I could not change, while learning, all over again, to trust Him.

With His love sustaining me, I kept trying to offer my beloved to Him. And, realizing what a long way there was to go, I tried to offer myself as well.

About a year after Dick was hospitalized, he seemed, again, to be walking about in a daze. I attributed it at first to the progress of the disease itself. Then I learned that he had a different doctor.

With the inevitable change of doctors in such a large hospital, it wasn't unusual that Dick's new doctor would prescribe the medication that he thought was best for him. He did, and with the same results as before.

Following the words of the well-known Serenity Prayer, "Give me courage to change the things I can," I protested (with explanation) to the director of General Health Care Services, himself an M.D. He immediately had the medication discontinued. Then he had a notice placed on Dick's chart stating that, thereafter, no psychotropic drug could be given without clearing through him, personally.

Such action was typical of the many things about that hospital that I came to appreciate. It was not only an efficiently run hospital, but a caring one, too.

During those months, there were ample opportunities to "accept" and to "offer up." There were countless other times when

I could do little more than cry out for God's mercy.

I had never wanted to give way to the often-heard lament, "Why me?" I had seen too much of the sufferings of others for that. So it was helpful when I read, about that time, that the pain we know in this life is but "a part of the human condition." Though that did not lessen my distress, it did much to strengthen my belief that we had not been singled out to suffer.

It was sometime that fall, after the drug had been discontinued, that I began to notice small changes in Dick—this time for the better. The first was when he greeted me one day with a happy smile as he called out, "Oh, there you are! I knew you'd come!"

I noticed that day that his pockets were full of rocks. The nurse explained that he had picked them up out in the courtyard—a lovely one with trees, shrubs and plenty of places to sit. Along with the dayroom it separated the wings for men and women. She said, yes, they encouraged such interests among the patients and, no, they didn't mind always having to empty his pockets.

Soon afterward, one of the aides spoke to me as I waited for them to bring Dick out, saying, with a twinkle, "You want to hear something cute?" Of course I said yes. "Would you believe that Richard is the only patient from the male ward who can wander down the women's ward anytime he wishes, and they love it! But just let any other man put his foot into their hall and they are told to get back where they belong, fast!"

Then she told me that the women patients called him "My Boy," and were very protective of him. This did not surprise me too much, for Dick had always had a gentle, somewhat innocent quality about him—now more than ever—and women liked to "mother" him.

When I asked how the men felt about him, if they disliked him, the answer was a laughing, "Oh, no! They call him 'My Buddy'!"

Then she went on to tell me how Dick had begun to laugh, clap his hands to music, and do little dance steps around the place. He brought many smiles to the patients and staff, who all delighted in him, she said.

A few days later, when I was signing the guest register, I heard some more of the same. The head nurse in charge of five buildings, of which Dick's was one, said to me as she looked up from her desk, "You know what we call him, don't you? We call him " 'Love'."

When I began to understand what a general favorite he had become, I remembered something long forgotten. I saw clearly the little white card, still stuck in the corner of the mirror of his dresser, which Dick had put there years before. Written on it were the words:

"Lord, What Shall I Do?"

I recalled how many times he had said he wanted to do "something special" for God. Often he had expressed the particular desire to work in a hospital so he could "help people." It would have been like him, I knew, to be willing to live—and die—in this slow and humbling way, if he could bring joy and cheer to others who needed it. He would have been glad, if in him they might feel a touch of God's love and gentleness.

To believe that God had permitted his illness for such a purpose would make it easier for me. For then, I could think of it as his ministry, and share the pain of it as we had shared everything else since first we met.

I had no way of knowing whether it really happened that way or not. But I did know enough of Dick's desire and intention to feel that I could offer it up to God for him. And I felt equally sure that God would receive the offering, and through this heartbreakingly slow disease, help him to continue to brighten the lives of those among whom he now lived.

"Hold him in the hollow of Your hand," I had always prayed for Dick. "Make him a blessing to others." I wondered if God, in His mysterious love, was but answering the prayers of Dick's heart and mine.

During the greater part of that year I felt as though we had been given a blessed reprieve. I began to feel that my part in all of it was to love him and to pray, and to accept Dick as he was and not as I wished that he might be. I determined to enjoy him as much as possible, as long as possible.

I found there was much left to enjoy. We walked on the grounds together, and fed "his birds" with nuts we had bought at the canteen. We went to the library, and though I was shocked to realize he could no longer read nor write, he enjoyed looking at pictures in the National Geographic and other nature magazines. We drove into Arcadia almost every week for shakes and hamburgers, which he liked.

Then there were the visits home which made him happy. We went for walks there—often several times a day—for he was very restless. Father Dage, our Curate from St. Luke's, came out each time he was home to bring him Holy Communion, and to pray for us both. I sometimes drove him over to the nursing home to see my sister.

Friends were good enough to come in and prepare dinner—especially when I brought him home for Christmas. For, since he had wandered away by means of an unlocked door one day, and was almost out of sight before I realized it, I knew I had to watch him every minute.

Back at the hospital, his group loved parties and we used any opportunity to give them one. Such an occasion was the time when several of Dick's Scout leader friends wanted to present him with an "Award of Merit" and a trophy inscribed with his name and "Palm District Distinguished Scouter."

The aides dressed him in his Scout uniform, which I had provided, and the presentation was made. He did not seem to understand what it was all about. But he did realize that something special was happening and delighted in the attention he was getting. He loved the party and even tried to help me in passing out refreshments.

It was that day that one of the women patients asked me, "Are you his wife?" When I told her I was, she asked, with a great deal of gravity, "Are you taking good care of 'My Boy'?" That was balm to my heart, for I rejoiced in knowing how much Dick was loved.

My heart was filled with thanksgiving that his life could still be, as I had always prayed, "a blessing to others."

Fourteen

Saying "Yes" to God

Retreat

O Lord, let this retreat
Be filled with Thy Spirit
Nor let me miss the faintest whisper
Of Thy love.

Oh, still my heart,
May I know the gentle touch
Of Thy dear hand
Turning me more surely
To Thy presence.

Attune my ear and my spirit
That I may hear
The ever so quiet strains
Of love's music
Singing to me.

Thy whisper, Thy touch,
Thy voice of tenderest love:
These I would perceive
With increasing clarity
That I may be drawn the closer
To Thy bosom.

With an ever-watchful eye over my beloved, I began to see that he was gradually growing more frail. I was startled and alarmed, however, when he became acutely ill with a bronchial infection and had to be moved to the Medical and Surgical Building—commonly called the "M. & S." This would be only the first of many times he would need to be there, for convulsions, blackouts, and various disorders.

This first real change, however, loomed large. It meant more adjustments for him and was thus distressing for me. I talked with the Director of Nurses, a devout woman of prayer who had become my friend.

"Richard's spirit is such a beautiful one," she said, "I don't think you need be too concerned about his adjustment. He seems to have a 'protective aura' about him that will keep him from being hurt." Then, gently, she put the direct question to me: "You do understand that you're going to have to lose him, don't you?"

I told her that I had lived with that fact for some time. Then I confided to her the prayer that was constantly in my heart: "Oh, God, You ordered our coming into this world. Please order our going out, according to *Your time, Your purpose* and the manner of *Your will*. Prepare us both for what is to come."

Even with that prayer, I had some misgivings. I loved Dick, and knew that I would miss him in this life. Yet, I wanted to be willing, and prayed that with God's help I would be ready, when the time came, to give him up.

For quite some time friends had been urging me to take some time to "get away." Always before I had resisted the idea, for I was reluctant to leave Dick.

But on a late afternoon in the fall of 1976, I found myself at All Saints Convent, just outside Baltimore. It was the first time that I had been away from him since he first became ill. I had come there with a special need.

Alone, that day, in my favorite spot on the spacious grounds, I watched the sun filter through the red and gold leaves of the maple trees, making a dappled pattern around me. Dick was very much in my thoughts.

Sitting there amid the beauty of All Saints, I realized how far apart we were—I, in Maryland, and he at the mental hospital in Florida. I relived the deep hurt of my recent visits with him, of yearning to see him, yet dreading, each time, signs of further deterioration.

It was a bit easier here, but soon I would be returning home. Not to the happy, laughing Dick I had loved, but to the now frail Dick, whom I loved even more, and who often looked at me with such soft, brown, puzzled eyes. Anguish gripped me. I seldom saw his ready smile—his look of fond recognition—except at rare and precious times like a flash of sun, peeping through a cloud. I thanked God, however, that he no longer understood what was happening to him and that, for the most part, he suffered no pain.

When I decided to get away for a while and my plane reservation was made, I had second thoughts about leaving him. I talked with one of the doctors about it. He said, "Mrs. Atkins, if he sees you today and tomorrow, or today and three weeks from tomorrow, it won't make any difference. He has lost all sense of time."

So, I didn't worry about his missing me. Nor did I fear for his well-being, knowing the love and care he received from those at the hospital. Gentle, dark-eyed Dolores, his charge-aide whom he loved, spoke for the others when she said one day, "Richard is such a dear. If all our patients were like him, our work would be cut in half."

As I reminisced, I thought of how I had prayed for Dick's healing from the beginning. I knew God was loving and that nothing was impossible with Him. Dick had always believed that, too.

I remembered how, as his illness continued, I had searched unceasingly for an answer in the Holy Scriptures, books on healing, healing missions and counselling sessions with those who led them. In God's mysterious providence, I learned, many are healed physically in answer to prayer, while others with a deep faith are not.

Slowly I had come to see more clearly what was meant by this "divine mystery," and knew that I must accept it. I did, and so began to pray, "Thy will be done in him." That prayer brought me a measure of peace that sustained me. At least it had sustained me until exactly two weeks before, when it had been so suddenly shattered.

It was when Dick's physician told me something that I'd never heard before. "Dick can live another twenty years or more," he said, "becoming as helpless as a baby—if not a complete vegetable."

I rushed from his office, distraught. "Not my Dick!" I wept as I ran for the car. "He's lost enough already—I can't bear to have that happen to him!"

Very troubled, I contacted Emily, whose spiritual judgment I valued so. "You must be willing for it to go on," she said. "Release him! Relinquish him! Offer him up to God for whatever period and for whatever purpose He chooses." In my grief and confusion, it was hard to grasp the full import of her words.

The continuing sense of distress and unease had prompted this trip to All Saints. When I had called Mother Virginia, the Superior, about coming, her understanding response was, "You just need to be refueled, dear." So, here in the silence, surrounded by love and prayer, I hoped to find an answer, some measure of serenity and direction.

"God, help me," I prayed that day under the trees. Please help me to understand." The quiet was broken, just then, by the Sisters' vesper bell. I arose and walked quickly up the path toward the chapel.

The next morning I returned, very early, to my hidden sanctuary. Little bits of sunshine sliced through the lacy green above me. I heard the wind's gentle whisper, and the birds—greeting the new day with their sweetest offerings. The world and its problems seemed far away.

Mine still lay in my heart and I prayed this would be the time when it would become clear. I felt God very near as I whispered once more, "Oh, God, please help me to see."

I can only believe that He did. For that day in my little hideaway at All Saints, I heard again those words: "You must be willing for it to go on. Offer him up . . . for whatever period . . . whatever purpose . . ." They took on new meaning for me.

For the first time I understood that always before, *my* "Thy will be done," had contained but two alternatives: physical healing or the spiritual healing of death. Though the latter had seemed to me the ultimate sacrifice, I had painfully reached a willingness to make it.

Now, questions began rushing into my mind, surprising me with their clarity. It was as though God spoke them directly to me. "But what of the other way? Are you willing to walk that path with him, for as long as I permit—accepting whatever comes?"

The simplicity and the enormity of those questions overwhelmed me. I recognized in them the real cause of my distress. It was simply a matter of trust! Did I trust Him, or not? Could I relinquish Dick completely, as I had so often been urged to do? Was I willing for it to go on and on? Could I say "yes" to the most difficult thing God had ever asked of me?

There, amidst those sacred environs, my answer came. I knew for a certainty that, with Christ, I *could* now say, "Let this cup pass, nevertheless, not my will but Thine . . ." And I did. There in the silence, I *had* to say "yes" to Him, for there was no other way.

It was not easy. My feelings were mixed at that point on Dick's journey, for it was *also my journey*, I knew. There would be pain, but with it God's peace—and loneliness, but always His love. Above all, I was convinced that each time I grew afraid, He would renew my faith, and strengthen me to endure.

St. Paul's words about endurance came to mind:

"Let us exult in our present sufferings, because we know that suffering trains us to *endure*, and endurance brings proof that we have stood the test, and this proof is the ground of hope." (Romans 5:3, 4)

While I did not understand, that day, all that was happening, I thought again of Dick's words to me, when he first learned what his future held. "Honey, we must be brave," he said. "We have to meet all these little trials and tribulations courageously, and just keep on going."

Once more, with God's help, I vowed to do just that.

Fifteen

Gift of Peace

Mystery Of Divine Providence

The mystery of Divinest Providence
stands towering o'er man's pinnacle of faith:

For Heaven's vaulted blue holds secrets rare
That mortal may not penetrate nor share;
We see but darkly now to run our race,
His promise: *then* it shall be "face to face."

Through all the pain and suffering of the world
man's offering whole—unfeigned trust in God:

To trust that we shall "know as we are known,"
That He will claim us wholly for His own;
Earth's veil will lift and mists dissolved shall be
As God reveals His *eternal mystery!*

It was almost two years since the spiritual struggle at All Saints, when I had said "yes" to God about Dick's condition—and really meant it. But I had learned that my "yes" required a continual, daily offering. Even so, the pain never went away.

I had kept on visiting him regularly. I also continued to bring him home at intervals, but saw each time further signs of his physical and mental loss. Worst of all, I watched as his loving communication slipped further and further away.

There was a time when he had greeted me with a happy smile saying jubilantly to the nurse, "Well, look who's here!" Or, "There she is!" But now his words were few, his eyes more shadowed and his manner alternately withdrawn and extremely restless.

In describing my distress to a friend, I said. "When I am with him, I have him—but I don't. He is with me—yet he isn't. I touch him and hold him and love him so, but feel that I have already lost him."

From the beginning, it had been a comfort to call and talk with Dick by telephone. In the early years, we talked several times a week—and then once or twice. Still later, the nurse or aide would take him to the phone and while he no longer talked, they said he seemed glad to hear my voice.

I remember well one particular day, and the pain (the sweet-pain) that my telephone call to him brought. I wrote down what I was feeling, for I never wanted to forget.

> God, why today?
> Why do I feel so lonely—
> Why do I hurt so much—
> Why do the tears insist on falling?

Today is no different
From any other day
When I miss him so—
Except . . . the nurse told me

That when I called him today,
His eyes were shining
And *he tried to kiss the phone*
When he heard my voice.

I kept on calling him as long as he seemed to respond, in even the smallest way, to my voice.

As time passed, there was less and less that we could share. Dick had always enjoyed going to the canteen. But now, though he was usually quite docile in going with me—would eat or drink whatever was put before him—the old animation was seldom there. His naturally joyous spirit was, more often than not, sadly lacking.

I kept on bringing him home overnight, but found it increasingly difficult to find anything that aroused a spark. He had always liked to have me play his favorite selections on the piano. But even in that, I no longer seemed able to reach him.

Burned into my memory is one particular time when I had brought him home for an overnight visit, a visit that would prove to be vastly different.

Though I took him out for walks several times, the locked doors (necessary because of his wandering) upset him more than usual. He tried the outside doors, one after the other. I kept calling to him: "Dick! Dick! Honey, come here with me. Oh, *please!*"

Nothing seemed to satisfy him. Nothing that I suggested could divert him from his preoccupation with the doors. He looked bewildered and distressed.

Finally, I had to face the question: If he is going to be this unhappy on his visits home, *why* do I keep bringing him? Is it for him, or for me? The answer was more obvious than I wished to admit, so I knew there was only one thing to do. I drove him back to the hospital that very afternoon.

On the way home with utter turmoil in my heart, I knew that my beloved Dick and I would never spend another night together.

Until that Saturday afternoon, several days after his shortened visit, I had not cried for a long time. In fact, I thought few tears remained. But that day, I felt low—physically tired, heartsick and lonely. The tears—unwanted and unexpected—kept getting nearer the surface. As I wandered restlessly from room to room, the silence became unbearable.

Finally, I rushed to the car, backed it out of the garage, and started driving—not thinking or caring about my destination.

Before long, I reached the outskirts of a small town called Lehigh Acres, about thirteen miles away. Without realizing it, I had headed straight for the community where Dick worked on a local newspaper his last eight years. I wondered at having come, for everything in sight reminded me of him.

I drove past the office where his friends were still working, past the theater where we had spent many enjoyable hours, and through our favorite shopping center. With each reminder the pain grew more sharp.

When the car finally came to a stop, I found myself at one of Dick's favorite spots. The lake was as round and sparkling as ever. The trees grew so close and so thick that it was hidden to the casual eye. Dick often liked to go there and take his lunch, so that he could sit at the lake's edge while he ate, feeding the squirrels and birds.

I could just see him sitting there, surrounded, as he so loved to be, by "God's little creatures." I could hear him, as he said, with his brown eyes shining. "Oh, they are so beautiful!" I remembered the special feeling he had for all living things. On the rare occasions when a large spider or a tiny chameleon found its way into our house, he would catch it and gently put it outside, saying, "Well, Honey, they're God's little creatures, too!"

Sitting in that silent place with only my memories, I put my head down on the steering wheel and wept unrestrainedly for the first time in a very long while. As I wept, there was the same unspoken prayer in my heart that had been there constantly during those miserable days since I had taken him back to the hospital. "Oh, Lord, I want to rest in You. I want to find peace. Please help me!"

Then I heard myself crying out loud: "Oh, God! I miss him so! I can't go on like this. Jesus, help me to find the peace You promised. Oh, God! *Help me!*"

When the tears finally began to subside, the prayers kept beating in my heart. Though I did not know it, the answer was nearer than I thought.

It was close to five in the afternoon when I drove away from the lake. On an impulse, I decided to stop at a nearby restaurant before returning home. At first, I was the only customer there. Soon an elderly couple came in. The man reminded me of Dick's father—

tall and thin and with the same friendly smile. The woman, short and plump, looked gentle and sweet, like his mother. I remembered Dick's Dad's death some years before, and his Mom's only recently.

Such thoughts brought an instant realization of the actual brevity of our life in this world. With that, my yearning for Dick and for God, all mixed up together, became so acute that I recall thinking (or saying), "Oh, God! If I could only see him whole once more!"

I was looking through a large picture window, at the time, toward the shimmering beauty outside, when the thought (or a voice?) came, "But, *you will!*"

With those words a strange thing happened. Everything around me seemed to become suddenly motionless—the waitress leaning over the old couple, a man across the street pedaling his bike, every leaf, every branch. Even the soft, white, luminous clouds ceased their movement in the sky. Each thing in sight appeared to be caught in a breathless state of suspended animation.

Though this silent and motionless scene seemed to last for a very long time, it could have actually been only seconds. But during that time, I found myself looking upon the whole muted drama as though I were outside or above it, seeing it from God's view rather than my own.

In a flash, I saw a strange similarity between life and a kindergarten class—how, in each, everything is real and earnest, yet so small. There came to me an awareness that our life on earth is something of a testing ground—a preparation, a prelude, to something infinitely more real.

Sitting alone in that small restaurant, I was bathed and flooded with a peace such as I have never experienced before. I knew that I would see Dick whole again. An unexplainable joy filled my heart as I glimpsed the difference between the transient and the eternal.

Whatever apprehension I felt concerning death left me. With new eyes I began to perceive that the most desirable of this world's offerings cannot compare with the beauty, the love, and the joy, that is to be ours. "Eye hath not seen, nor ear heard, neither has entered into the heart of man the things which God has prepared for those who love Him." (11 Cor. 2:9)

I knew, that for one brief moment, I had been given a fleeting glimpse into the "eternal mystery."

I went into that restaurant in tears. I left with the joy and peace of a loving and compassionate God. I shall never forget what happened there.

Sixteen

The Spirit is Living and Well

No Earthly Fetters

The sadness is but sad to me
  He walks unknowing in the light—
    No earthly fetters left to bind
His spirit as he walks with Thee.
    Oh, grant me valiantly to fight
      That joy with Thee, I too, may find.

For quite some time I had suspected, as had those who worked with him at the hospital, that Dick was not able to see well. There was no way we could tell whether it was the result of the Alzheimer's or whether a change of glasses might help.

When he began running into things, we knew that something needed to be done. The hospital made appointments and sent him in their van, with a nurse, first to one ophthalmologist and then another. Two had brain wave machines. One was unable to test him, he said, because he couldn't "focus his eyes," the other, because he couldn't "report back what he saw."

With great concern, I finally called the head of the Wilmer Eye Institute at Johns Hopkins in Baltimore. After explaining Dick's problem to him, I said, "I'll fly him any place in the United States if I can find help for him."

The doctor answered, "Fortunately, Mrs. Atkins, you won't need to fly him very far. Your husband needs what is called a retinoscopy, and one of the best doctors in the country for that is Dr. Jonathan Trobe, at the Veterans Administration Hospital's Medical Eye Center in Gainesville, Florida." And so here we were, once more, on our way to Gainesville.

The small plane sped steadily forward, slicing through the rolling, white clouds before us. From my seat beside the pilot, I turned to look at Dick, who was directly behind me, with the registered nurse on his left. Satisfied that he was all right—he looked more alert than usual, though not afraid—I looked ahead again. It was easy, with only the drone of the plane breaking the silence, to let my thoughts drift back over the events of the past year or so, and to the more recent cause of our being where we were at that moment.

In my reverie, that July morning in 1980, much came back to me. I remembered how, when I could no longer keep Dick overnight, I had kept on taking him home for a part of a day, even though doing so meant a total of 180 miles of driving.

Then I thought of the time when he had fallen during one of his convulsions and knocked out some front teeth. Though the hospital dentist said a permanent bridge wasn't feasible, I had to be sure; and took him to three dental surgeons in Fort Myers, only to hear the same thing. In his condition—and in the light of his serious reaction to drugs they all agreed that administering the necessary anesthetics was too risky. The only alternative—soft food.

Then I remembered when Dick started having blackouts. Each time, he had to be rushed to the M.&S. building by ambulance, on a stretcher and with oxygen. A shot had to be administered to bring up his blood pressure, which always plummeted to a dangerous low.

It was after he had suffered several such blackouts that I was strongly advised against taking him home anymore. "Mrs. Atkins," the doctor said, "If he had one of these blackouts on the way home, and didn't get the help he needed immediately, he could die sitting right there beside you."

Just thinking about it caused me to turn and look at the nurse and the little bag beside her. It was comforting to know that Dick's hospital had supplied her with a syringe and the medication needed in case he should have a blackout on the way. I started to speak to Dick but noticed he was half asleep, and so patted his knee instead.

As the plane droned on, I thought of all the planning that had gone into this trip, and the people who had helped—especially the doctors and nurses at G. Pierce Wood Hospital. I was thankful for them, and also for the Air Ambulance Service, called Air Trek, and the Personnel Pool from which I had gotten the name of the kind nurse who now sat next to Dick.

And then there was Merve—Father Mervin Allshouse—who had driven us to the airport that morning in my car and would meet us when we returned. I had a warm feeling when I thought of Merve. He and Dick had been friends while working with Boy Scouts, long before he went to seminary, and before Dick's illness began. During the past six or seven years, especially since Bishop Haynes had appointed him vicar of St. Edmund's Mission in Arcadia, he had provided inestimable support to us both. Regularly, each week, he had met me at G. Pierce Wood and brought us Holy Communion. He always had special prayers, not only for Dick, but for me. I sent up a quick prayer of thanksgiving as I asked God's special blessing upon him.

Before I realized it, the pilot glided to a stop. We were in Gainesville.

During the forty-eight hours we were in Gainesville, I had spent most of my time at the Veterans Administration Hospital, going to my nearby motel room only to sleep. Just that morning the doctor had given me the results of all Dick's testing. "Mrs. Atkins," he explained, "his visual pathways are almost perfect. But due to the Alzheimer's, he is unable to process the image he gets." Then he continued, "I believe he will be able to see well enough to get around as long as he can walk. But I predict that he won't be walking a year from now."

That my heart was heavy at such dire news was understandable. But despite the heaviness, I felt a small measure of peace, because I knew everything possible had been done for him. There was nothing more I could do.

Merve met the plane and drove us back to the hospital. After we left Dick, I told him what the doctor had said, he was as grieved as I. We agreed that it was just one more thing that we had to accept and offer up to God. To offer it not only for Dick, but for others who suffered, we felt would be a very special kind of intercession. We both knew that Dick would have been glad for that.

Though Dick had always enjoyed our little jaunts into Arcadia, those, too, had to come to an end. When we took him into town on his birthday that October to get a haircut and have dinner at the hotel, we decided not to try it again. His knees had become so stiff that it was with great difficulty that we managed to get him into and out of the car. Merve, my next-door neighbor who had gone with us that day, and I agreed that it had become too hard for him.

As the months passed, I saw other changes taking place in Dick. Very early in 1981, I said to Father Dage one day, "He seems to be moving further and further away from me."

His understanding reply was, "But remember, for every step he takes away from you, he is one step closer to God."

It was about that time that I heard a bishop say that only if we suffer willingly can we have a share in Christ's Passion. He pointed out that our Lord never said, "Follow me and I will give you an easy, painless path through life." But that His poignant message was, "Follow me, choose the same way of life as mine, and I will give you a share in my suffering."

Almost as if on cue, in the last week of July, 1981—exactly as Dr. Trobe had predicted—Dick finally lost his sight; and almost simultaneously, had to go into a wheelchair. Through the deep hurt, I prayed that God would bestow upon him spiritual wholeness and make him a continued blessing to others.

In his frailty, his was still a gentle spirit. My heart rejoiced each time I was told that his life had blessed, in some small way, that of another—often one who lovingly cared for him. More than once a nurse or an aide would express the sentiment, "I wish I could have known Richard when he was well. You can just tell what kind of person he must have been."

It was easy to see, in that devastating disease, the steady decline of Dick's mind and body. I felt sure, however, that only God could fully see his spirit. I was convinced that He not only saw, but was holding the spirit of my loved one in His most tender care.

One look into Dick's face reflected not a mindless existence, as some have called it, but the "calm and patience and peace of his nearness to God" to quote one of his nurses.

It brought me comfort, many times over, to be able to say of Dick, and believe it, *"The spirit is living and well."*

Seventeen

Letting Go

Relinquishment

The slow paced journey shortens
    as he goes from me to Thee
In his final embarkation on the
    vastness of life's sea.
Relinquishment of him, O Lord,
    to Thy love's sweet embrace
I cannot make, except for mercy's
    requisite of grace.
To release him to that "Larger Life"
    that now awaits him there—
Unfettered by my human strands of love
    is now my prayer.
Oh, grant that I not hold him at Thy call:
    "My child . . . now come,"
Nor cling in grief, when in his love
    his answer leads him "home."
Oh, give me of Thy courage, gather up
    these waves of pain,
That my love's last offering for him
    reparation may attain.
Oh, summon him in Thine own time, but
    be gracious, Thou, to me . . .
From dark to resurrected light, let me share
    Thy Calvary.

The year, 1982, did not start out well at all. Dick had been quite ill during the holidays. In mid-January I received a letter from the director of General Health Care Services. It expressed the same compassion for Dick and me that I had learned was typical of those who worked at G. Pierce Wood Hospital. It said, in part, "This is to advise you that Richard has improved sufficiently to be removed from the list of our seriously ill patients. However, he is not completely out of danger. Relapses are frequent and serious. At the present time, however, the improvement is a hopeful indication and we are happy to advise you of this . . . . With diligent nursing care, medical care and prayer, we are hopeful his improvement might continue . . . . Be assured that all is being done to accomplish Richard's recovery, and we will keep you advised as to his progress."

"Relapses are frequent and serious." This proved to be all too true. I never knew, when I drove up to see Dick, whether he would be in his own building or in a skilled care ward of the M. & S. building.

He developed a very serious skin disorder which kept him there a good part of the time. At regular intervals he was sent to a dermatologist in Port Charlotte, a town some distance north of Arcadia. He was transported by van, on a stretcher, with a driver and usually two aides. I drove up each time he was there to be with him.

That spring, during one of his worst bouts with this distressing malady, a couple from out of state came to see him. They and he had been very close friends since childhood. I appreciated their faithfulness in visiting him, for they came every year, without fail. I knew that it could not have been easy for them—especially this year. But they always hoped—and so did I—that he could understand that they were there.

I will never forget a card they sent me once, which I cherished. On the outside the printed message said, quite simply, "Your sorrow is our sorrow." Inside, written by hand, the words: "It *truly* is." I knew how much they meant it.

During the summer, Dick had a longer than usual period free of serious illness. I took advantage of that time to fly up to All Saints—my favorite place—for a time of rest and "refueling," and to do a bit of writing.

When I told Mother Virginia of the precarious condition of Dick's health, she told me the Sisters prayed for us both daily, and urged me to "commit him to God." Then she expressed a beautiful thought which lifted my spirits. "No amount of everlastingness on this earth," she said, "will ever make up for the quality marriage you and Dick had." Since she had met Dick on several occasions before his illness, her words were all the more meaningful to me.

Upon my return from All Saints I saw that Dick continued to grow more frail. As the months went by, I felt an increasing inability to cope with it all.

Of course, through the years, there had been many times of feeling "down," but none of them ever lasted. I had shed tears on countless occasions, but usually felt better for having done so. I had suffered over every loss I saw in Dick, and the pain never really left me. But through it all, God had strengthened me and enabled me to "accept" and to "offer him up." So why, I wondered, is it different now?

Perhaps it was because my husband had been ill more than usual that year. Perhaps it was because *I* had been hospitalized twice in a period of months. Perhaps it was because there was so little communication left between Dick and me, and I was missing it so. Perhaps the heart attack my sister had suffered, serious enough for me to be asked to come to the nursing home in the middle of the night, played a part. Or, perhaps it was just that, over the years, I had grown so very, very tired. I simply had no answer.

Since the early days of Dick's hospitalization, there had been those who assumed that because he was in a mental hospital, I must be in a state of deep depression. I had resented that assumption, and fought against such stereotyping as I continued on with my life in as normal a fashion as possible. But I knew enough about the signs of real depression, to see, at that point, that there was cause for concern.

I was more sad then ever, crying at every little thing, feeling more lonely than for a very long time. I found myself pleading with God, over and over, for help. I could not seem to rise above my despondent feelings. For the first time in the almost fourteen years of Dick's illness and his eight years in the hospital, I felt that I couldn't—and wasn't sure that I *wanted* to go on.

This lasted for a month or two, or perhaps three—I don't quite remember. I only know it kept getting worse. Then, a very unusual thing happened. I do believe in the Communion of Saints and have heard people say that after their loved ones died, they seemed so near at times, and to be of comfort to them. But, of course, Dick was still living. Yet . . . but let me go back a bit.

At my lowest ebb I decided to seek help from a priest–psychologist of our diocesan counseling service, who spent one day a week at our parish, St. Luke's. I had talked with him only once, several years before, when I just happened to be there on his day. I recalled his telling me then that he didn't think I needed any deep therapeutic counseling—just someone to talk with now and then. At that time, Father Dage and I often talked. He was not only a friend and a caring priest, but his wife's mother had suffered from Alzheimer's, which made him particularly understanding of our circumstances. But he had been out of the state for more than a year and a half.

When I saw the counselor, I told him how desperate and depressed I felt. Then I said, much to my own surprise, "I think I know what the problem is."

"Tell me about it," he prompted.

"Well, when I think of Dick, the pain is just *too* sharp. Yet, when I try to put my mind on other things—to turn my thoughts away from him—I feel as if I am deserting him."

His reply was quick and to the point, "In other words, you are laying a guilt trip on yourself that you neither need nor deserve."

I had never thought of it like that. We talked on for a while, about that and other things, and made arrangements to meet again in two weeks.

It was during that interval that a very extraordinary happening took place.

Of course, I was doing a lot of praying all the while. Then, suddenly one day, I realized that it was as if Dick was walking beside me, encouraging me. It seemed that I could actually hear him speaking, in words like these: "Honey, don't worry about me, I'm all right." Or, "You must go on with your life—your writing and the other things, God wants you to do." And, "Please, try not to be sad. Try to trust in God. He knows what He is doing.''

Over and over I heard him. And the strange thing was, though it did not seem at all strange at the time, I answered him—out loud: ''Yes, Honey, I'll try.'' And, ''Yes, Dick, I will, I promise!''

This unusual dialogue continued for four days and nights. I have never really understood it, nor do I expect anyone else to do so. I only know that it happened.

It was during that time that God gave me a special prayer poem, which could only be called ''Letting Go.'' If anyone had asked me, during all those years of Dick's illness, if I had let him go, I would have said ''yes.'' I thought I had. But I began to see clearly that the one way I had never let him go was in my thoughts. Praying that prayer brought me the kind of peace that I had never experienced about him.

> O gracious God,
> Grant that I may no longer try
> to hold him in my mind
> Nor yet endeavor
> to turn thoughts of him
> away.
> Help me
> to let him come and go
> at will:
> In coming, to find a loving,
> welcoming prayer
> And in going, a blessing
> as soft as sweetest air.
> But, Oh!
> In leaving him free
> to enter or to leave my mind
> Do Thou lock him in my heart
> and hold us both in Thine,
> That he may ever be
> a part of me
> And we, O Lord . . .
> of Thee.

When I saw Father Harrison the next time, I told him what had happened. After we discussed it and he read the poem, he said, ''I don't believe you need me any longer.'' He went on to say, however, that if at any time the load got too heavy, to call him and we could talk.

That whole experience—whether I understood it or not—was a

wonderful one for me, and one I shall never forget. It did not mean that the loneliness was gone, nor the restlessness at the life I was forced to live. It did not mean that the pain of watching Dick's increasing helplessness grew less. But it did mean that the despair that had been wrapping itself so slowly and relentlessly about me completely disappeared.

I knew that it was God who had mercifully delivered me. And for that, I was deeply thankful.

Eighteen

*God's
Mysterious
Ways*

Life's Fullness

The air is crisper and the green is greener
When the heavens its rain has shed,
And the stream struggling over the rocks is grateful
When its emptiness has been fed.

If our empty soul and our struggling spirit
Could but know what all Nature knows—
We would lift our eyes and look to the Source
From Whom all of life's fullness flows.

And knowing that He is both Source and Supply
Of the blessings poured over our head,
We can drink of the fountain of Living Water
As we wait by Him to be fed.

Then our hearts will lift up in sheer gratitude
To this Source of life, Who is God . . .
And we'll joyfully trust Him *all the way*
As we follow the Path He has trod.

With the encouragement of interested friends, I decided to attend a Christian Writers' Conference held in Nashville in the summer of 1983. My interest in writing went back a way, but during the past few years it had helped to fill many lonely hours.

I had been encouraged as more of my poems appeared in periodicals and anthologies. Some articles were printed under my name, and a short story brought the first actual monetary reward.

A book of meditations, though bringing quite good comments from a number of publishers, had not found a taker. When I learned how difficult meditations are to sell, especially by an unknown writer, I set it aside, hoping for better success in the future.

At the conference, my spirits were lifted and my will strengthened to keep on writing. I only wished that I could share it with Dick; he had always been so proud of my least endeavor.

After leaving Nashville, I planned to visit my nephew and his family in Memphis. The wait in the airport gave me ample time to call the hospital and check on Dick.

I called and reached his social worker, who had become a good friend of mine. She assured me that there was no noticeable change—that, for him, Dick was doing well. I felt relieved to hear that.

"Marguerite . . ." she hesitated.

"What is it?"

"I don't know whether you've heard, but, Father Allshouse died yesterday. I'm so sorry. I know how much he meant to you and Richard. We will all miss him around here."

After the conversation was over, I sat waiting for my plane with a saddened heart. I remembered the last time I saw Merve. It was in the Venice Hospital, the Tuesday before I left. He had known for a long time that he had leukemia, but the doctors had been able to keep it fairly well under control. But when he came down with a severe case of pneumonia, that was not so easy.

When I had been allowed in to see him, he was glad and so was I, for he had proved himself a true friend. Soon after I arrived, a retired priest came to give him Holy Communion. And invited me to join Merve. I did not know that it would be my last time to receive with him, but will always be grateful to have been there.

After the priest left, we talked. Merve was in a very good mood. I didn't want to tire him and started several times to leave. Each time, he would say, "Oh, you don't have to go yet—it's a long time till dark," (He knew I had a distance to drive and needed to get home before night.)

We talked, naturally, of Dick and of many other things that day. He told me that he might retire when he left the hospital, but said not to worry. He would have even more time to spend with Dick then.

It was a good visit and I shall always cherish the memory of it, and of him as a real friend and man of God.

On my way to Memphis that day, there was a mixture of feelings in my heart. I knew how he would be missed by his family, and my heart lifted in prayer for them. He would be missed, also, by many others who knew and cared for him.

I knew that I would always miss him, and his loving support. Many times over, I had realized that when he was there for my visits with Dick, I never went home quite as tired. His presence, his humor, and his caring way with Dick had always been very special. Whether he was helping me lift Dick when he slipped down in his wheelchair or pushing him when we took him outside, or just talking so lovingly to Dick, calling him "Buddy," I knew it would never be the same without him.

And who would bring us the Holy Sacrament week by week, lay his hands on our heads and pray? He had cared so much. A feeling of great loss swept over me. How could I possibly manage with Dick, without him?

I knew there would be other patients at G. Pierce Wood who would miss Father Allshouse too, for the priest at St. Edmund's usually acted as chaplain to the Episcopalians who were there.

Then I thought of St. Edmund's itself, and how this would leave them without a priest, and I wondered who would be sent to take his place.

Just thinking of St. Edmund's brought back many pleasant

memories. In the early years after Dick and I moved to Fort Myers, his parents lived in Winter Haven and my sister in a nursing home in Tampa. Our favorite way of traveling to either place took us through Arcadia.

I don't remember when we first discovered that lovely little church, but we did. Thereafter, we always stopped on our way home, usually late Sunday afternoon, for a short visit. We had agreed that the quiet peace—the almost palpable atmosphere of prayer—was what drew us to the altar rail and held us there while we prayed.

After Dick was hospitalized at G. Pierce Wood, only seven miles away, we continued to visit St. Edmund's almost every week. In the early years, Dick knelt with me at the altar rail. As his knees began to stiffen, he would stand beside me, as I knelt, and hold my hand. He always seemed more peaceful after we had been there. Then the time came when he was no longer able to go.

I knew I would always love that little church. I prayed that our Lord would help the Bishop to choose the right priest. Since St. Edmund's was small and classified as a mission instead of a parish, I knew the responsibility would be his.

———————

"God works in mysterious ways" is a phrase that many of us have heard from childhood. I had not only heard it but had, on numerous occasions in my life, seen proof of things happening that could have been accounted for in no other way.

Usually these had been instances in which God had answered specific prayers of mine, or of someone else. But I was soon to see how God, with one clearly defined action, could answer the prayers and meet the diverse needs of many.

This is how it happened: Father Dage and his family had been out of the diocese of South West Florida for about two years when they felt they should return. Though he had no church to come to, they came back anyway praying that God would guide them and show them where He wanted Father Dage to be used.

The first time I saw him after his return, he said to me, "I'm sure God has a plan for us, but He hasn't let me in on it—*yet.*"

They had been invited by Merve Allshouse' son and daughter-in-law to stay with them for a few weeks in Fort Myers. (They had been friends when the Dages were at St. Luke's before.) That would give Father Dage time to talk with Bishop Haynes and to learn of any possible openings in our diocese.

It was only natural, then, that he went, on several occasions with Merve's son to visit his father in the Venice Hospital, and to take him the Holy Sacrament. The bishop asked Father Dage to act as supply priest at St. Edmund's while Father Allshouse was in the hospital.

The people liked him so much that, after Merve's death, they requested the bishop to send him to St. Edmund's as their priest, and he did.

When I returned from Memphis, I heard the good news. Father Dage had been appointed Vicar of St. Edmund's, and that meant he would be the one to visit Dick and bring him the Holy Sacrament. I was grateful, for I had not forgotten how he had ministered to Dick in the early years of his illness, whenever I brought him home.

How like God, I thought, to answer so many prayers and to meet so many needs by this one action! I realized anew how He was both source and supply of this and of all our blessings.

Father Dage and his family were happy with the appointment, as were the members of St. Edmund's. Bishop Haynes, I felt sure, was glad to fill the vacancy with one who had already proven himself in the diocese. And I couldn't have been happier if God had asked *me* to make the choice!

That didn't, of course, mean that Merve would not be missed, but rather, that he would want God's work to go on. Father Dage put it very well when he said that Father Allshouse had laid a good foundation, upon which he would be priviliged to build.

I could only marvel at "God's mysterious ways," as did others. Prayers of thanksgiving ascended, I am certain, from countless hearts besides mine.

Nineteen

All the Way

Life's Mysteries

Life is filled with small mysteries
Like the sun setting through the leaves,
The fields that are bare and empty
When the farmer gathers his sheaves,
The light that fades at the end of day
Bringing night when we cannot see
Or the pain that comes when we're alone
And long with a loved one to be.
Then there is always the face of death—
Our own or that of a friend—
When in grief, for a time, we wonder
If death in this life *is* the end.

But surely as the crimson sun descends
We know it will rise in the morn—
The hours of darkness flee away
When a beautiful day is born.
And, as in the emptiness of the field,
A new crop replaces the old
We often find that our loneliness
Is filled with the purest gold.
So shall we see at the end of life
Its final, sweet mystery:
A door that opens through death to new life
With God . . . in Eternity!

It was well after midnight when the telephone rang. With a feeling of apprehension, I hurried to pick up the receiver.

"Hello."

"Is this Mrs. Atkins?"

"Yes, it is."

"Mrs. Marguerite Atkins?"

"Yes."

"Wife of Richard Atkins?"

With my heart beginning to pound, I once more answered in the affirmative.

"I am calling from G. Pierce Wood Hospital—and I'm sorry, I'm sorry to tell you . . ."

My heart was beating furiously, and my feeling of alarm was so great that I cried out, "What's wrong? Tell me. Is Dick ill, or is he *dead*? Please! Tell me!"

It was then that the resident chaplain told me that my beloved Dick had died suddenly in his sleep, less than an hour before.

I remember crying out, "No! Oh, no!"

"The doctor would like to speak with you, Mrs. Atkins."

I was so shaken that I heard only a few of the doctor's words —something about "a regular bed check," and "cardiac arrest." When he began to ask a few routine questions, I was unable to answer. I promised to call him later.

At my request, a friend came over to stay with me for a while. I called the doctor back, and immediately afterwards, called Karen.

A few moments later, Father Dage telephoned from Arcadia— the chaplain had contacted him. It was good to hear his voice. One thing that he said still stands out clearly in my mind. "Marguerite, I want you to remember one thing."

"What?"

"Remember that Dick is not ill any longer—he is whole." I understood what he meant, and it comforted my heart to hear him say it.

Not long after he hung up, I had a call from Father Ryan, my Rector from St. Luke's. Father Dage had telephoned him. He expressed his deep sympathy and assured me that he would be glad to help in any way that he could.

Finally, after the telephone calls were over and my neighbor had returned home, I locked the door, turned off the lights and went back to bed, but not to sleep.

My thoughts were a jumble; they skipped from one thing to another. I had known he was going to die, but not like this—so suddenly. "Oh, God," I cried, "why does it hurt so much?" I had seen for years how steadily he was going downhill, and remembered how happy it had made me when someone spoke of it as his "transformation, not deterioration."

Then I thought of the doctor who had said, only two weeks after meeting him, "That's one beautiful man!" At the time it warmed my heart. But after he lost his sight and went into a wheelchair, his smiles had all but disappeared.

He hadn't talked much after that, either. There was that one last time, more than two and a half years before, when he surprised me by responding with more than one word. I was rolling him out the door into the sunshine one day, when I leaned over and said, "Honey, you know I love you, don't you?"

His answer was as clear as it was unexpected, "You know I know."

At the thought of it, I buried my head in the pillow, as I cried, "Oh, Darling, I'll miss going to see you and touching you, and doing things for you! I'll miss hearing you say, "I . . . love!"

For the last year and more his spoken responses had been few. Sometimes, when feeding him something that he had always liked, I might say, "Is it good?" Over and over I would repeat the same question. Finally, as if with great effort, he would say, ". . . Good!"

Or, I would say, repeating the same words many times, "Honey, I love you. Do you love me?" If I kept saying it long enough he would invariably answer, "I . . . I *love!*"

I had felt that perhaps his hearing was impaired until one wise and experienced nurse had offered another possible explanation. "Perhaps it takes him that long after you first ask the question to gather together all the resources at his command to answer you."

One part of me felt bereft. Then, in my memory I saw him again, as he was before the illness began—with the smile on his face and the laughter in his eyes. I felt the tenderness of his touch.

With that, memories of things past filled my mind. I thought of how, soon after our marriage, he said his first grace over our meal. It was so real and like him, that I urged him to continue, which he did as long as he was able. I still use it. (My friends know it as "Dick's grace."):

"O God, we thank Thee for this food. Bless it so it will give us strength, courage, love, health, and more understanding of Thee, and of other people. Amen."

Thinking of him that night, I saw again the joy that had been such a part of him, his zest for life, the enthusiasm which caused me sometimes to say laughingly, "You're just a Peter Pan! You'll never grow up!"

His usual quick and impish reply was: "Who wants to grow up? That's no fun!"

But with all his lightheartedness, he had a more serious side. The Scout laws were deeply meaningful to him, and he lived them every day. Whether trustworthy, helpful, kind, brave, reverent—or any one of the others—all had become an integral part of his nature. He lived as well, his obligation to the Order of the Arrow: "To be unselfish in service and devotion to the welfare of others."

I had wondered at times about his loyalty to scouting, his love for St. Francis of Assissi, and his deep commitment to our Lord and His church. Where did one leave off and the other begin?

My conclusion, long since, had been that they didn't. They had become, rather, a mature blend and a totality of all that Dick was. And I wondered that night, Isn't that what a Christian's life is meant to be?

Amidst such thoughts of him, the stark fact that he was gone suddenly intruded again. But with my spirit I knew that he was gone only from my sight, and I felt thankful that he was free from his infirmities.

Then, just as suddenly, there came into my mind something that had taken place only a few weeks before. Some of us had felt that Dick had a "flash" of sight occasionally, though we couldn't be sure. Even so, I was totally unprepared for what happened that day.

I was waiting for him when the aide brought him out of his ward at the end of the hall. When he was about six feet away, he seemed to look straight at me, and his face broke into a beautiful smile. I couldn't believe it! I hurried to him and greeted him joyfully as I gave him a warm hug. It had been more than two years since I had seen him smile like that!

His social worker had stepped out into the hall just in time to see what happened. "You can't make me believe that he didn't see you just then!" she exclaimed.

During the entire visit that day, his eyes followed me, and his happy mood continued. It brought joy to my heart, even though I did not understand it. It never happened again. But my heart holds dear the one time it did.

As I lay in my bed, I wondered if it were possible that our merciful Lord had granted me that one joyful time as Dick's last, loving, earthly gift to me.

In between the tears shed that night, and all the remembrances, my heart finally found its deep core of peace. I recalled how Emily had said so many times that it is God Himself, and not healing for healing's sake, that we must seek above all else—that the spiritual healing always supersedes the physical.

I believed that to be true. And as the first streaks of dawn began to appear, I knew beyond any doubt that Dick was with God and that he had, at last, received God's spiritual healing. I gave Him thanks as I sank into a brief but peaceful sleep.

The "waiting" between Dick's death and his funeral was made easier by the kindnesses of friends, and particularly by the presence of my nephew, Pat, from Memphis, and Karen, from Ohio. Pat spent some time with my sister at the nursing home, and he did numerous things for me that really mattered. It was a special comfort to have Karen for several days, for we have always been close. She is so very much like her father!

Monday evening we had a short "visitation" at the funeral home. I knew the real Dick was not there—that his spirit was with God—but I had not seen him since the Wednesday before, when he had looked strangely distressed. A hint, perhaps, of a tired heart which would last only a few more days? Of course, we do not know.

Karen wanted to look upon her father's face once more, also. We were both glad that we had done it, for he looked as peaceful as in the years before his illness began.

I was doubly glad when, very unexpectedly, Bishop Haynes walked in. He had come from St. Petersburg for a meeting and had driven a considerable distance out to the funeral home to see me. It was good to feel his warmth and his caring, as he prayed for the repose of Dick's soul, and then prayed for me.

———————

The funeral, at St. Luke's Church, was beautiful. Father Ryan conducted a Requiem Mass, assisted by Father Dage. It was strengthening to receive the Holy Sacrament at such a time. Though not at my peak of concentration, parts of the scriptures and prayers that I had requested stood out for me.

"For I reckon that the sufferings of this present time are not worthy to be compared with the glory that shall be revealed in us." (Rom. 8:18) And, from the fourteenth chapter of the Gospel of St. John, the well-loved words: "Let not your heart be troubled . . . I go to prepare a place for you . . . that where I am, there you may be also."

One verse from St. Francis' prayer was so meaningful that Karen and I agreed that it should become a part of the permanent marker over Dick's grave: "In dying, we are born to eternal life."

At the conclusion of the service, Father Dage read aloud a poem which had a special significance to me. It was one about Dick, which I had written the summer before at All Saints, and had called "All the Way." In February, it had been accepted by *The Living Church,* a weekly Episcopal magazine, to be published "sometime in the future." In God's providence, that "sometime" was September 11th, 1983, just six days before Dick's death.

> He is my loved one,
> But Thou didst create him
>   and so lovest him more.
> I know Thou wilt be near him
>   in his illness . . .
> Thou wilt hold him close in Thy arms
>   as a mother cradles her child
>   while sleeping.
> Thou wilt bear him up, and
>   carry him gently on his journey
>   all the way.

Those who knew how Dick had died, so gently in his sleep, were deeply moved, as was I. That God did love him, hold him close and carry him gently *all the way*, I have no doubt at all. Nor do I doubt that He answered my constant prayer to "order Dick's going out" according to His time, His purpose, and the manner of His will.

I cannot close this chapter or this book, without saying that, yes, there have been tears—for I miss him—and the pain has not all gone away. But there is in my heart, as well, a deep joy and thankfulness that my loved one has found *wholeness* at last. I can pray for him now, in the sure knowledge that he prays, also, for me.

To go to G. Pierce Wood Hospital, to play the hymns for a monthly service in the chapel, as I do, is not depressing to me at all. Rather, I feel a warmth toward all who cared for him with such devotion. Being there helps to keep me reminded that he is no longer imprisoned by his physical body, nor subject to earthly ills.

I see Dick now, as his own joyful self, but with the added radiance which comes from being among the "saints in light." (Col. 1:12) I am convinced that *he is with God, who loves him, and who loves each one of us* (as He promised) *with His "everlasting love."* (Jer. 31:3)

Epilogue

Say "Yes"

I sat in a dimly lighted church
Where at first I could not see;
In love and in hope I waited
For Thy Spirit to come to me.
Alone, in that sacred, hallowed place
The darkness began to clear
And the vigil light reminded me
That Thou art *always* near.
I lifted to Thee a questioning heart:
'O Lord, what shall I do?'
The answer came in tones most sweet,
"Say 'yes' when I ask you to."

I've willed, dear Lord, to say "yes" to Thee
Since that moment so long ago
When first I said it with sorrow,
For the one whom I've loved so.
Thou knowest his heart belonged to Thee,
That it never wavered, when
He learned of the illness he must bear
Until his life should end.
But now, tonight, my loved one is gone,
Called in his earthly sleep—
Borne on angels' wings, I know,
His tryst with Thee to keep.

All praise, Blest Lord, for holding him close,
As I so oft did pray,
And for Thy dear love, in carrying him
So gently . . . *all the way.*

(Written two weeks after Dick's death)

157

About Alzheimer's Disease

Editor's Note:

The following article is based on information supplied by two leading neurologists, Dr. Melvin Greer, Professor and Chairman of the Department of Neurology of the College of Medicine at the University of Florida in Gainesville, Florida, and Dr. Douglas A. Newland, a member of the Neurology Associates of Lee County in Fort Myers, Florida. We also drew extensively on literature supplied by the Alzheimer's Disease and Related Disorders Association, Inc., (ADRDA), located in Chicago, Illinois. To all three sources, who gave so generously of their knowledge, we extend our thanks.

Alzheimer's disease is the fourth leading cause of death in the United States. Although the illness can occur in the forties and fifties, it more typically strikes older age groups—five percent of all persons over 65 and ten percent of those over 80. Today, almost two million older Americans suffer from Alzheimer's disease, and this number is increasing. Says Dr. Newland, "Advances in medical science are helping to conquer heart disease, stroke and cancer, allowing people to live long enough to develop the incurable Alzheimer's."

The disease was first described in 1906 by a German neurologist, Aloise Alzheimer, who recognized certain microscopic patterns in the brains of its victims. In Alzheimer's disease, the nerve endings in the outer layer of the brain degenerate so that electrochemical signals cannot pass between cells. These areas of degeneration can be seen under a microscope and are known as plaques. Other changes visible through autopsy are accumulations of tangled fibers. The larger the number of these two abnormalities—plaques and tangles—the more devastating the impact on the brain's "executive actions"—memory, emotion, and higher intellectual functioning.

Yet despite Aloise Alzheimer's findings almost 80 years ago, the notion of "hardening of the arteries" as the major cause of senility has, until quite recently, persisted. It is now known that approximately 50 percent of older persons suffering from severe mental impairment have Alzheimer's disease. About another 25 percent have diseased blood vessels and the remainder a variety of other conditions, such as brain tumors, thyroid dysfunction and pernicious anemia. Since Alzheimer's disease is virtually imperceptible in its early stages, and in any event, its symptoms mimic many other —usually treatable—conditions, diagnosis is not a simple matter. Says Dr. Greer, "The physician who examines the Alzheimer's patient in the early stages may not be able to detect any abnormality unless indepth neuropsychological testing is carried forth."

Although the clinical course of Alzheimer's disease varies— ranging from two to 20 years and often including periods of normal functioning—a distinct progression is apparent. In the early stages, family members may notice subtle changes in the individual's behavior—loss of memory, withdrawal, irritability and difficulty in mastering organized motor tasks. As the disease advances on its tragic, relentless course, thinking processes become so impaired that the sufferer must depend wholly on others for survival. Problems with personal hygiene, disorientation and sleep disturbances are frequent, as are psychiatric disorders—depression, paranoia, and aggressive outbursts. In the final stages of the disease, deterioration of the brain is so widespread that the person is rendered "mute, inattentive and paralyzed."

What causes Alzheimer's disease? "Heredity and age play a crucial, but unexplained role," says Dr. Newland. "Aluminum toxicity, head injuries and ultra-small infectious particles are other unproven theories." To date, many treatments have been tried, including the injection of a chemical substance directly into the brain, but none have met with any real success. Research continues, but for now, Alzheimer's disease cannot be cured or prevented.

What, then, can be done to help the person who develops this disease? "Treatment of the patient includes primarily supportive measures," says Dr. Greer. "By that I mean the understanding of the family to help the patient live as an accepted member of society." For the patient who withdraws from family life, Dr. Greer recom- mends gently encouraging him or her to participate, while being careful to keep this coaxing at a level that will not induce additional stress. Aggressive behavior can sometimes be changed by removing the individual to a calmer place, away from the source of agitation, says Dr. Greer. For problems with motor function, such as buttoning clothing or tying shoelaces, he advises encouraging self-help but only to a degree that will match the person's capabilities.

Family members taking care of the person afflicted with Alzheimer's disease should learn all they can about the symptoms and progress of the disease. From the beginning, the patient should be under the care of a physician, who can monitor the progress of the disease, answer the many questions that arise, and treat other ailments that may complicate the course of Alzheimer's disease.

A valuable source of support for caregivers is the Alzheimer's Disease and Related Disorders Association (ADRDA), which is made up primarily of the families of persons stricken with Alzheimer's. Its purpose is to raise public awareness, provide support to families, and gain financial support for research. ADRDA has more than 100 chapters and affiliates, along with 300 family support groups throughout the country. A listing of ADRDA groups in any particular area may be obtained by writing to their national headquarters at 360 North Michigan Avenue, Chicago, Illinois, 60601.

The battle against Alzheimer's disease, sometimes called the "silent epidemic," has only just begun. As dedicated medical and scientific researchers, health care professionals and support organizations work to gain a better understanding and perhaps one day a cure for this tragic disease, there is hope for its victims and their anguished families. And there is comfort, too, for in reaching out to one another through support groups, these families know that they do not suffer alone.

64422